Heart Smart

The Women's Guide to Heart Health and Stroke Prevention

By
Well-Being Publishing

To You,

Thank you!

Table of Contents

Introduction:
Empowering Your
Heart Health Journey

Embarking on a journey to improve heart health is a courageous and necessary step towards longevity and well-being. Heart disease remains a leading concern worldwide, especially among women, who often experience unique symptoms and risk factors. This book serves as a comprehensive guide to understanding heart disease, learning its intricate impact on the women's body, recognizing warning signs, and embracing lifestyle strategies to foster a stronger, healthier heart.

Heart health is not merely about avoiding illness; it's about empowering yourself to live a life full of energy, joy, and vitality. It's about making informed choices that not only prevent and manage heart disease but also improve the overall quality of life. This journey you're about to undertake is rooted in education, motivation, and actionable solutions that will transform the fabric of your daily existence.

The human heart is a marvel of nature, a symbol of life and emotion. To protect it, we delve into the anatomy and functionality of the heart, especially focusing on how it relates to women. Understanding how your heart works sets a solid foundation for grasping how lifestyle factors like diet, exercise, and stress management directly influence its health.

Recognizing the signs of a stroke, a formidable adversary of heart health, is critical. This book will arm you with knowledge and protocols to respond swiftly should such an emergency arise. In parallel, we will examine common risk factors that each individual has the power to control. Smoking cessation, diabetes and cholesterol management, and maintaining an optimal weight and blood pressure are all signposts on the path to a healthier heart.

Yet, some elements lie beyond our grasp. Genetics, family history, age, and the natural course of menopause - these are the risk factors we cannot change. However, our approach and response to these chal-lenges can define our heart health narrative. This book encourages a proactive stance, guiding you to seek wisdom over worry.

Nutrition plays a pivotal role in heart health. A heart-smart diet isn't about restriction; it is about embracing wholesome foods that nourish and protect. You'll learn about heart-boosting nutrients, decipher myths surrounding fats and sugars, and discover how to make dietary choices that invigorate your cardiovascular system.

An active lifestyle is essential for a robust cardiovascular system. Exercise is not a one-size-fits-all endeavor, and we will help you tailor a fitness regimen that strengthens not just your heart, but your entire self. Cardiovascular and strength training exercises are your allies, ready to fortify you against heart disease.

Your mental health is just as important as your physical health when it comes to your heart. Stress, left unchecked, is a silent saboteur of cardiovascular well-being. Techniques like mindfulness can break the cycle of stress, leading to a more harmonious existence between heart and mind.

Navigating the healthcare system and understanding heart health tests can seem daunting. Your journey will be guided by insights on selecting healthcare providers, understanding essential screenings, and staying proactive in your relationship with medical professionals. Knowledge is power, and in healthcare, it becomes your strongest advocate.

For those living with heart disease, there's a spectrum of support and information available to enhance recovery and quality of life. Discussions around rehabilitation, medications, and tapping into emotional and social support networks provide a blueprint for thriving post-diagnosis.

Prevention is the cornerstone of heart health. Adopting lifestyle choices that favor cardiovascular health and engaging in regular screenings create a defensive shield against heart disease. Your daily decisions wield the power to shape your heart's destiny.

As you read through the chapters, you'll also discover heartwarming stories of strength, survival, and hope. These narratives are not just tales; they're evidence of human resilience and the victories possible when equipped with the right knowledge, tools, and spirit.

Your heart-smart future awaits. It's a journey that demands consistency, awareness, and an unwavering commitment to oneself. Let's embark on this transformative voyage together, where each step taken is a step closer to a healthier heart and a fuller life.

To support your journey, we've included comprehensive resources, heart-healthy recipes, and versatile exercise guides that cater to all fitness levels. And finally, a glossary of heart health terms will decode medical jargon, making the science of heart health accessible to all. So let's begin this empowering journey for your heart, for your health, for your life.

Chapter 1:
Understanding Heart
Disease in Women

As we turn the page from our introduction and embark on a transformative health quest, Chapter 1 calls upon us to delve into the heart of a critical topic: heart disease in women. Often misunderstood and misdiagnosed, heart disease claims countless lives yearly, yet its hold on women presents with particular intricacies. Whether you're a health professional or someone grappling with heart disease firsthand, an astute understanding of how it uniquely affects women is pivotal. Bridging gender-specific gaps in knowledge and awareness can lead to life-saving prevention, diagnosis, and treatment strategies. We'll uncover the layers of heart disease and strokes specific to women, emphasize risk factors that target the female population, and spotlight symptoms that should trigger immediate action. As we lay the groundwork for a heart-conscious lifestyle, let's unite in recognizing the silent nuances of women's heart health, their profound importance, and the undeniable strength within every woman's reach to combat the unseen adversary.

Defining Heart Disease and Stroke

Understanding heart disease and stroke is the crucial first step in your health journey. Envision a complex highway system, where every road, bridge, and pathway is vital for transporting necessary supplies to a bustling city. Much like this network, your cardiovascular system—

including your heart, veins, and arteries—supports your body's every function, every moment of your life. Heart disease encompasses a range of conditions that affect this intricate system, leading to inefficiencies or blockages in the blood flow, much like traffic jams or collapsed bridges would interrupt a city's operations.

At the heart of these conditions is coronary artery disease (CAD), the most common form of heart disease. CAD occurs when the major blood vessels that supply your heart with blood, oxygen, and nutrients become damaged or diseased. Cholesterol-containing deposits, known as plaques, and inflammation are usually to blame for this narrowing and blockage that characterize CAD, drastically affecting heart function. It's essential to comprehend that heart disease is not a single entity but a collection of problems that afflict the heart in various ways. This understanding can empower you to seek specialized care and adopt targeted lifestyle changes to address your specific condition.

Another condition falling under the heart disease umbrella is heart failure—a term that understandably strikes fear into many. However, equipped with knowledge, one can counter its progression. Heart failure does not mean the heart has stopped working; rather, it is struggling to pump blood as well as it should. Factors like high blood pressure or previous heart attacks can leave the heart too weak or stiff to fill and pump efficiently. Recognizing and managing these underlying causes can be life-changing and life-extending.

Atrial fibrillation (AFib) is a heart rhythm disorder that is often highlighted in discussions about heart disease. With AFib, the heart's upper chambers (the atria) beat chaotically and out of sync with the lower chambers (the ventricles). This irregular rhythm can lead to blood clots, stroke, heart failure, and other heart-related complications. And while AFib may sound intimidating, awareness, and prompt treatment can make it manageable, allowing one to lead a full and active life.

In the most literal sense, a stroke is an attack on the brain, much as a heart attack is an attack on the heart. This attack comes in different forms—the most common being ischemic stroke, where blood flow to the brain is blocked, often by a blood clot. Hemorrhagic stroke, less common but more deadly, occurs when a blood vessel in or around the brain bursts. Strokes can lead to significant disabilities or death, but with immediate attention and intervention, the damage can be limited.

The notion that heart disease and stroke are men's issues is a dangerous misconception. In fact, women often endure unique risks and symptoms, which can lead to misdiagnosis or delayed treatment. The challenge is intensified given that women's heart disease symptoms might be subtler or different than men's. For instance, during a heart attack, women may experience shortness of breath, nausea, and fatigue, rather than the classic chest pain.

Understanding the intersection between heart disease and stroke reveals the vital importance of vascular health. These conditions share common risk factors, such as high blood pressure, high cholesterol, smoking, diabetes, obesity, and physical inactivity. Moreover, these factors can be addressed, to a significant extent, through lifestyle choices that you have the power to make. Empowerment lies in the understanding that your day-to-day decisions can dramatically impact your risk and your quality of life.

Early detection and management of heart disease play an extraordinary role in improving outcomes. Regular screenings and being in tune with your body can catch issues before they escalate into crises. Embracing a proactive approach towards heart health can make all the difference—it's about making small but consistent choices that prioritize your wellbeing, which accumulate into a robust defense against heart disease and stroke.

When we talk about stroke, we must also discuss the importance of urgent medical response. Recognizing the signs of a stroke quickly and accurately can save your life or the life of someone you love. The faster one acts, the better the chances of minimizing brain damage and potential long-term disability. By understanding and spreading knowledge about the symptoms and the immediate actions required—through protocols such as 'FAST' for face drooping, arm weakness, speech difficulties, and time to call emergency services—you become an active participant in the fight against stroke.

Advances in medical technology and treatment strategies have dramatically improved the prognosis for individuals with heart disease and stroke. Interventions such as stents, bypass surgery, and medications can alleviate symptoms, prolong life, and enhance life quality. However, it's crucial to remember that these medical interventions work best when complemented by a healthy lifestyle.

Discovering how to live with heart disease includes learning about the conditions themselves. Knowing the difference between stable angina (chest pain that occurs with a predictable level of activity or stress) and unstable angina (chest pain that occurs at rest or with minimal exertion) is just one example of the specifics that can guide your treatment and lifestyle adjustments. Education is a key tool—it builds confidence in managing your condition and encourages communication with your health care team to tailor a plan that fits your unique situation.

It's imperative to recognize that you're not alone on this journey. Heart disease is a widespread challenge, affecting millions; your story is part of a larger tapestry. Embracing a community—whether it's support groups, online forums, or connecting with others who share your experience—can offer strength and insight. Through shared experiences, you can find solace and strategies to cope with and overcome the emotional and physical hurdles that heart disease can present.

A heart attack, or myocardial infarction, presents yet another facet of heart disease. It occurs when a part of the heart muscle doesn't receive enough blood. The severity of a heart attack can vary greatly, from a minor incident that serves as a wake-up call to a life-threatening event. Whether it's your first or a subsequent heart attack, it's life-changing. This clarity is a beacon, guiding you to a path where every choice—from diet to exercise, from stress management to sleep—becomes a part of your healing and a pledge for your future.

In the context of strokes, understanding and preventing second or multiple strokes is crucial. The lifestyle changes and medications used to treat a stroke are also integral in preventing further strokes. Here lies an opportunity for transformation. Whether it's embracing a new diet rich in fruits, vegetables, and whole grains, or integrating physical activity into daily life, every positive change is a step in building resilience against future cardiac events.

Ultimately, defining heart disease and stroke is not just about understanding medical terms and conditions. It's about comprehending the implications on your life and recognizing the power within you to influence your health trajectory. With knowledge as your ally and deliberate, informed actions as your tools, you can shape a journey toward heart health that is proactive, hopeful, and life-affirming.

Risk Factors Unique to Women

When we seek to understand heart disease, it's essential to recognize the unique risk factors that affect women. These nuances in health and wellness enhance our strategy for prevention and management of cardiovascular conditions in women. Let us delve into the aspects that shape a woman's journey through heart health.

Hormones play a significant role in the heart health of women. Estrogen, commonly referenced for its role in reproductive health, is believed to offer some degree of protection against heart disease. However, as women approach menopause and estrogen levels decline, this protective effect diminishes, potentially increasing the risk of developing heart issues.

Pregnancy-related complications, such as gestational diabetes or preeclampsia, are not only immediate concerns but can also indicate heightened risks for cardiovascular disease in the future. Women who experience these conditions should closely monitor their heart health with their healthcare providers.

Autoimmune diseases, which are more prevalent in women, such as rheumatoid arthritis and lupus, are connected with an increased risk of heart disease. Inflammation caused by these disorders can contribute to the buildup of plaque in the arteries and other heart-related issues.

Mental health is intricately linked with heart health, and studies have shown that depression and anxiety disproportionately affect women. The stress these conditions induce can lead to high blood pressure and other heart risk factors. Consequently, it is vital to include mental well-being as part of a comprehensive approach to heart health.

Polycystic ovary syndrome (PCOS) affects women's endocrine system and is associated with a cluster of conditions that elevate heart disease risk, including insulin resistance, increased blood pressure, and elevated cholesterol.

The atypical presentation of heart attack symptoms in women often leads to delays in seeking treatment or misdiagnosis. Unlike men, women may experience less recognized symptoms, such as jaw pain, nausea, or fatigue, which can mask the true cardiovascular nature of their condition.

Women are more likely to have microvascular coronary disease, a condition that affects the smaller arteries in the heart. This condition can be more challenging to diagnose and treat effectively, consequently carrying a higher risk of debilitating heart issues.

Lifestyle factors, while affecting both sexes, can be particularly insidious for women. Metabolic syndrome — a combination of fat around the abdomen, high blood sugar, and high blood pressure — develops differently in women and has been linked to higher cardiovascular risks.

Women often play the role of caregiver, balancing careers with family commitments. This can lead to high levels of stress, which is known to exacerbate heart disease risk factors such as hypertension and obesity.

Contraceptive methods, which may include hormones, can introduce an increased risk for blood clots and high blood pressure. The compounding effect of smoking and the use of hormonal birth control further raises the heart disease risk in women significantly.

Breast cancer treatments, including radiation and chemotherapy, can affect the heart, and survivors need to be aware of long-term cardiovascular monitoring and management.

Iron deficiency and anemia, which are more common in women due to menstrual blood loss and childbearing, can lead to an increased heart rate and eventually heart enlargement and heart failure if not properly managed.

Understanding the social determinants of health reveals that women, particularly in underserved communities, are more likely to face barriers to healthcare. Lack of access to proper nutrition, healthcare services, and health education can all contribute to the increased risk of heart disease in these populations. It's imperative to address these disparities in order to provide equitable heart health prevention and care.

In conclusion, these women-specific risk factors demand tailored approaches to prevention, diagnosis, and treatment. Healthcare providers should be attuned to the nuances of assessing heart disease in women, and women themselves should be empowered to know and understand their unique risk factors. By embracing a proactive stance, integrating lifestyle adjustments, and seeking informed medical care, women can effectively manage their heart health and mitigate their risk of heart disease. The journey is deeply personal, but with knowledge and support, it becomes a pathway to a healthier heart and a fuller life.

Symptoms Women Should Never Ignore

As we delve deeper into understanding heart disease, it's vital to address the warning signs that demand immediate attention, especially within the female population. Women's heart symptoms sometimes differ subtly from men's, and recognizing these nuances can literally make the difference between life and death. With each beat, your heart sends life-preserving blood throughout your body; in return, it's only fitting that you pay close attention to what it might be trying to tell you.

Let's first discuss chest pain, a hallmark symptom of heart trouble. While men often report a crushing or severe pain, many women experience this sign as a pressure or tightness—a sensation that can be mistakenly attributed to non-cardiac causes. It's imperative not to dismiss such symptoms, particularly if they're accompanied by discomfort in the neck, jaw, shoulder, upper back, or abdomen.

Shortness of breath, another critical symptom, can emerge in instances lacking physical exertion. This feeling, as if you can't catch your breath or you're gasping for air, can signal heart problems, especially if it comes on suddenly and unexpectedly.

Inexplicable fatigue or weakness, which could surface days before a heart attack, also warrants attention. If you find yourself feeling unusually tired, even after adequate rest, or if you encounter sudden exhaustion while performing activities that used to be easy, it's time to consult a healthcare professional.

Next, palpitations, described as the sensation of skipped heartbeats or a fluttery feeling, can be a clue. While often benign, it's important not to ignore palpitations, especially if they're accompanied by other concerning symptoms.

Nausea or indigestion are signs often shrugged off by many as related to less serious digestive issues. However, if these symptoms persist without an apparent cause and are paired with any of the heart distress signals mentioned earlier, they should not be taken lightly.

Sweating or cold, clammy skin that occurs without physical exertion or exposure to high temperatures might indicate a stress response due to cardiovascular strain. The body's attempt to cool down in the absence of external reasons could hint at an underlying heart condition.

Lightheadedness or sudden dizziness, particularly with simultaneous chest discomfort or shortness of breath, must be regarded as a red flag. This can, at times, precede fainting and should prompt you to seek medical evaluation promptly.

Unexplained symptoms that seem to appear predominantly during physical activities—like climbing stairs or carrying groceries—can also be signs of heart disease. If these activities become more difficult due to symptoms like those described, it's a profound signal that your heart might be struggling.

In the context of heart health, leg swelling or edema, though common in various conditions, should ring alarm bells if it occurs without a reasonable explanation. This symptom could indicate heart failure, especially if it's accompanied by shortness of breath and fatigue.

Persistence of symptoms is another important consideration; transient discomforts are often less concerning than those which are relentless or increasing in intensity. Your body's consistency in signaling discomfort is a way it communicates the urgency of the situation—do not ignore it.

Quietly and dangerously, heart diseases can masquerade as other ailments, leading to misinterpretation and delay in treatment. Stress the importance of staying attuned to your body's signals and maintaining an open dialogue with your healthcare provider regarding any unusual symptoms.

Moreover, during pregnancy, postpartum, and throughout menopause, women should be particularly vigilant. The physiological changes during these times can increase the risk of heart problems, making it crucial to pay heed to any unusual symptoms.

Embrace the power you hold over your health. By recognizing and responding to your body's distress calls, you're taking a pivotal step in protecting your heart. Your health is a priceless asset—don't devalue it by overlooking symptoms. Proactive steps and responsiveness to your body's warning signs are instrumental in safeguarding against advancing heart disease.

In conclusion, while some of these symptoms could have benign causes, the stakes are far too high to take chances with your heart. Understanding your body's language is not only empowering—it's essential. The vigilance you maintain today can secure the wellness of your heart tomorrow. When in doubt, always err on the side of caution and consult with a healthcare professional. It's your life, your health, and your heart at stake, and each moment of mindful attention can help to ensure a future of vitality and longevity. In the next chapters, we will continue to explore the anatomy and function of the heart, as well as strategies to maintain its health, but always remember that immediate attention to worrisome symptoms is the cornerstone of cardiac wellness.

Chapter 2:
The Heart of the Matter:
Anatomy and Function

Embark on a transformative journey into the core of your wellbeing as we delve into the intricate world of your heart's architecture and its vital role in sustaining life. Understanding the heart's anatomy and function is foundational to grasping the essence of cardiovascular wellness and preventing the cascade of changes that lead to heart disease. The heart is not just a biological marvel—it's a muscular powerhouse, diligently pumping life through your body with synchronized beats that fuel our every move. It's a labyrinth where electric impulses signal the tempo, valves ensure a unidirectional flow, and arteries and veins form an expansive highway of nourishment. As you come to appreciate the relentless work of this extraordinary organ, you'll be equipped with the knowledge that's crucial for recognizing the early signs of distress and navigating the steps you can take to ensure its longevity. This chapter aims to illuminate the intricacies of your heart's design, shedding light on its relentless rhythm; a beat keenly attuned to the demands of your body and life. This understanding is the first step on the path to a resilient heart—one that's supported by lifestyle choices that echo its steadfast nature.

Exploring the Female Cardiovascular System

The heart beats, unmistakably essential, propelling our existence forward with every rhythmical thump. Woven into the fabric of life, the cardiovascular system's purpose is both powerful and delicately intricate, especially within the female form.

Anatomically, the heart and vascular system are comparable between men and women, yet distinct differences mark the female cardiovascular system. Structurally, women's hearts are generally smaller, and the layers that make up the wall of the heart, known as myocardium, are thinner. Smaller coronary arteries equate to different manifestations of heart disease and varying symptoms. Please keep this architectural uniqueness in mind as it influences everything from clinical symptoms to the mechanisms of heart disease and its treatment.

During the course of a woman's life, she experiences specific physiological shifts that can influence the health of her heart. Notably, the hormone estrogen plays a seemingly protective role in maintaining flexible arteries and facilitating healthy blood flow. However, as a woman transitions into menopause, estrogen levels decline, often leading to changes in blood vessels and an increase in cardiovascular risk. Understanding this transition is critical for prevention and early detection.

Women's cardiovascular health can exhibit distinct symptoms, challenging both diagnosis and intervention. For example, while men may experience the classic symptom of chest pain during a heart attack, women might face subtler signs such as fatigue, shortness of breath, or jaw pain. Recognizing these nuanced symptoms is vital for prompt and appropriate medical attention.

Moreover, the electrical activity of the heart, which orchestrates its rhythm, can present variations between men and women, influencing conditions such as arrhythmias and the side effects of medications. It's not simply a matter of scale; the gender-specific physiology requires gender-specific medical considerations and approaches.

The connection between pregnancy and cardiovascular health can't be overlooked either. Conditions such as preeclampsia and gestational diabetes are not only concerns during pregnancy but can also serve as harbingers of future cardiovascular issues, indicating the need for ongoing heart health monitoring postpartum.

Regarding lifestyle, women often take on multiple roles and responsibilities, which can influence heart health through the pathways of stress, time constraints on exercise, and dietary choices. Creating balance and establishing heart-healthy habits are actionable steps women can take to nurture their cardiovascular system amidst life's endless demands.

Stress is not some abstract concept when it comes to your heart; it's as palpable as the blood coursing through your veins. For women, it's essential to acknowledge the unique stressors they face and understand how these stressors can tighten the grip on their heart health. Mind-body connection strategies, including mindfulness and relaxation techniques, can serve as a bastion against the siege of stress.

Preventive strategies are a linchpin in maintaining cardiovascular well-being, particularly for women. Regular physical activity tailored to a woman's life stage can enhance circulation, manage weight, and keep blood pressure in check, collectively acting as a keystone of cardiovascular resilience.

Dietary considerations also have a gender-specific component. Understanding the interplay between diet, hormonal balance, and cardiovascular health informs the choices you make three times a day. Nutrient-rich diets that include elements such as fiber, healthy fats, and antioxidants can help modulate inflammation, which is believed to play a pivotal role in the development of heart disease. It's more than simply eating well; it's about fueling the very essence of your heart's health.

When considering medical interventions and medications, women must be discerning consumers of healthcare. Treatment protocols that are gender neutral fail to embrace the intricacies of the female cardiovascular system, which can lead to less effective outcomes. Partnering with healthcare providers who appreciate these complexities and advocate for women-specific research is key.

As we delve deeper into heart health, we must cultivate an awareness of the female cardiovascular landscape—a terrain marked by both vulnerability and enduring strength. There's a profound beauty in transforming knowledge into empowerment, allowing women to advocate for themselves with conviction in the pursuit of optimal heart health.

As the narratives of heart disease continue to evolve, women must be at the forefront of rewriting their script. No longer sidelined by data skewed toward male physiology, women are staking their claim in the heart health domain, demanding recognition of their physiological uniqueness and the tailored care they deserve.

Your heart's health shines as a beacon that illuminates every area of your life. By attending to it with the care it demands, you harness the potential to not only extend your years but also enrich the quality of every moment. The process is one of enlightened self-care—forged not only in the crucible of shared experience and scientific insight but also in the intimate knowledge of your body's narrative.

As the awareness of women's heart health gains momentum, let it be a tide that raises all ships. Whether you're a health-conscious individual, a concerned caregiver, or an adept healthcare professional, you play a role in the grand symphony of heart health. Together, through persistent education, advocacy, and prevention, we can craft a future where women's cardiovascular health is not only explored but exalted and preserved for generations to come.

How Heart Disease Develops Over Time

Understanding the progression of heart disease gives us the power to influence the trajectory of our health. In its earliest stages, heart disease can be subtle, beginning with risk factors such as unhealthy diet and physical inactivity that might not immediately show any symptoms. Over time, these behaviors can result in the accumulation of plaque in the coronary arteries — a condition known as atherosclerosis.

Atherosclerosis is often the root of heart disease and doesn't appear overnight. It builds gradually, often over decades. Initially, this plaque build-up may not disturb the blood flow to your heart. However, these deposits can harden and narrow your arteries, leading to decreased blood flow, or in more severe cases, complete blockage.

Chronic inflammation plays a pivotal role in this progression. Whether due to lifestyle factors or underlying conditions, inflammation can damage the arteries, making it easier for cholesterol to deposit in the vessel walls. This not only accelerates plaque formation but can also make existing plaque unstable. When plaque ruptures, it can trigger the formation of blood clots, which can potentially lead to a heart attack or stroke.

Blood pressure and cholesterol levels creep up over time, often a byproduct of lifestyle choices and sometimes genetics. As blood pressure rises, the heart has to work harder to pump blood through the body, which can lead to the heart's walls becoming thicker and less flexible. This condition, known as hypertrophy, can further exacerbate heart disease progression.

As heart disease advances, the heart muscle can become damaged or weakened. This can result from inadequate blood flow due to narrowed or blocked arteries or from the strain of chronic high blood pressure. Eventually, this damage can lead to arrhythmias, heart failure, or other heart disorders.

Beyond the physical changes, heart disease can influence other body systems. For instance, reduced blood flow can affect kidney function, which may lead to fluid retention and strain on the heart. There can also be a significant impact on the brain, as heart disease is a risk factor for cerebrovascular disease, leading to cognitive decline or stroke.

Subtle signs often go unnoticed, such as shortness of breath, fatigue, and decreased stamina, which can initially be attributed to aging or lack of fitness. This highlights the importance of regular health check-ups as they play a key role in early detection.

Menopause brings an additional risk for women as changes in hormone levels can affect cholesterol and blood pressure, accelerating the development of heart disease. While younger women generally have a lower risk than men for heart disease, this risk equalizes and can even surpass that of men as women age.

Despite the gradual nature of its development, heart disease can suddenly manifest through an acute cardiac event, like a heart attack. This is commonly the first indication for many that they have heart disease, which underscores the insidious nature of its progression.

Modifiable lifestyle factors are the most influential aspects of heart disease progression. Nutrition, physical activity, smoking cessation, and stress management can have profound impacts on the development of heart disease. Taking proactive steps in these areas can slow or even reverse some of the damage, showing that the heart has a remarkable ability to heal if given the right environment.

While we can't change our genetic blueprint, understanding our familial health history can help us take preemptive actions. Knowing what we're up against empowers us to prioritize heart health and potentially alter our health destiny.

Progression doesn't mean inevitability. Even those who have experienced a heart event or surgery can find new hope and opportunity for healing. The heart's plasticity allows for new pathways and improved blood flow, often resulting from lifestyle changes and medical interventions that can lead to a hearty recovery.

In conclusion, the importance of recognizing how heart disease develops over time cannot be overstated. By acknowledging both the silent nature of its progression and the power we have to change its course, we set the stage for proactive, preventative, and potentially life-saving strategies. Embrace the role you play in your heart's health—your future self will thank you for the care and attention you invest today.

Chapter 3:
The Silent Killer: Recognizing
Stroke Signs

As we delve further into the complexities of heart health, it's vital to pivot our attention to strokes—a formidable adversary in the fight against cardiovascular disease. Recognizing the harbingers of this silent killer can mean the difference between life-altering damage and full recovery. Strokes spare no time; they strike swiftly and without mercy, making it imperative to understand and identify their signs promptly. Knowledge is power, and in this chapter, we empower you with the lifesaving information needed to discern the subtle and overt symptoms of a stroke. Acting quickly isn't just advisable; it's essential. Just as a seasoned warrior anticipates their opponent's next move, you can learn to anticipate the signs of a stroke—the numbness in the limbs, the sudden confusion, the loss of balance—and respond with the urgency needed to minimize its impact. We're not just aiming to inform; we aim to inspire you to take immediate action at the onset of symptoms, potentially saving precious brain cells and preserving the quality of life. Through this vital knowledge, you stand guard over your health and well-being, ready to confront one of the most formidable foes of heart health with confidence and wisdom.

Types of Strokes and Their Impact

A stroke occurs when blood flow to an area of the brain is interrupted or reduced, preventing brain tissue from getting oxygen and nutrients.

The effects of a stroke can be long-lasting and vary depending on the part of the brain affected and the amount of tissue damaged. But did you know that not all strokes are alike? There are several types of strokes, each with varying causes, treatments, and potential impacts on health.

Ischemic Strokes - are the most common, accounting for about 87% of all strokes. They occur when blood vessels become narrowed or blocked by clots, drastically reducing blood flow to the brain. Ischemic strokes carry profound implications: they can cause permanent brain damage, disability, or even death if not promptly treated.

Hemorrhagic Strokes - happen when a weakened blood vessel ruptures and bleeds into the surrounding brain. This type of stroke is less common but much more deadly than its ischemic counterpart. It's a stark reminder that managing high blood pressure can be a matter of life and death, as it's often the underlying cause.

Transient Ischemic Attacks (TIAs), also known as mini-strokes, are short-lived, displaying similar symptoms to a stroke but typically resolving within 24 hours. Though they may seem less severe, TIAs should be taken seriously—they are often a warning sign of a future stroke.

The impact of a stroke is not merely physical. Cognitive functions, such as memory, attention, and the ability to solve problems, can be significantly affected. A stroke can also have emotional consequences, such as depression or anxiety, creating a ripple effect that extends to loved ones and caregivers.

The areas of the brain impacted by a stroke often determine the nature of the consequences. For instance, a stroke in the brain's left side can hinder speech and language capabilities, whereas a stroke in the right side might impair spatial and perceptual abilities. The cerebellum's affliction can disrupt balance and coordination, whereas the brainstem's involvement might impair vital functions like breathing and heart rate regulation.

It's critical to recognize that the duration of symptoms can help identify the stroke type. For example, if symptoms vanish within 24 hours, a TIA is likely. Yet, lasting symptoms indicate a more severe ischemic or hemorrhagic stroke. Prompt medical response is paramount in both scenarios.

Recovery from a stroke hinges on immediate treatment and the nature of the stroke itself. Post-stroke rehabilitation can be a lengthy process, involving physical therapy to regain movement and strength, speech therapy to recoup communication skills, and occupational therapy to sharpen everyday abilities.

Secondary prevention is equally crucial following a stroke. This involves the rigorous management of risk factors such as high blood pressure, atherosclerosis, atrial fibrillation, and diabetes. It's a proactive step to stave off another stroke and underscores the importance of lifestyle changes and medication adherence.

The psychological impact can't be overstated. Support groups and counseling may play a significant role in a patient's recovery, aiding them in dealing with the emotional aftermath of a stroke, which may include grief, frustration, and anger.

Furthermore, strokes can lead to medical complications that extend beyond the initial event. Challenges can include difficulty swallowing, which can lead to malnutrition or pneumonia, or develop into more chronic conditions such as limb spasticity or urinary incontinence, which can profoundly affect a person's quality of life.

Understanding the different types of strokes and their implications allows for targeted interventions. Knowing that certain drugs can dissolve clots in ischemic strokes or that surgical options exist for hemorrhagic strokes can influence treatment plans significantly.

Education can empower individuals to recognize stroke symptoms early. Quick action can dramatically alter the course of recovery, underscoring the importance of public awareness initiatives and the value of knowing the FAST (Face, Arm, Speech, Time) protocol, which will be discussed in the next section.

The impact of a stroke extends beyond physical and cognitive damage—it's a transformative event that can change a person's life and identity. The aftermath of a stroke isn't just about survival; it's about learning to live a new life with new challenges and opportunities for growth. With the right support and resources, recovery and adaptation are possible, but the key lies in prevention and awareness.

Each individual's journey following a stroke is unique—some may experience rapid recovery, while others may face a lifelong process of adaptation and rehabilitation. However, the common thread is resilience. With the advancing stroke care technology and a deeper understanding of rehabilitation, individuals have greater chances of regaining independence and quality of life than ever before.

As we move forward, remember that the fight against strokes is multifaceted. It begins with prevention through education and lifestyle changes and continues with providing swift and decisive care during a stroke. Rehabilitation and support round out the battle, helping survivors find their footing in the aftermath. Awareness of the types of strokes and their impacts puts power in our hands—power to act, to prevent, and to regain control after a stroke has occurred.

The FAST Protocol for Stroke Response

When it comes to heart health and mitigating the risks of stroke, knowledge truly is power. The FAST protocol stands as a sentinel, a quick and easy-to-remember method to identify the early signs of a stroke and act immediately. Understanding what each letter signifies can make a life-saving difference not only for those at risk of heart disease but for anyone who may witness someone experiencing a stroke.

F in the FAST acronym represents Facial drooping. One of the most visible signs of a stroke can manifest as an asymmetry in the face. Ask the person to smile; if one side droops or doesn't move, this could indicate that a stroke is occurring. Recognizing this symptom promptly and responding can vastly improve outcomes.

A stands for Arm weakness, where an individual may be unable to raise both arms and keep them elevated due to weakness or numbness in one arm. This could be another clear indicator of a stroke, given the lack of muscle control resulting from a neurological impairment that requires prompt attention.

The third component, S, is for Speech difficulties. When someone's speech becomes slurred or they seem unable to express their thoughts coherently, it's time to be concerned. This highlights the potential impact of a stroke on areas of the brain associated with language and communication.

T embodies Time, underscoring the importance of immediate action. Time is brain, as medical professionals often say. The chance of recovery and minimal brain damage diminishes with each passing minute during a stroke, making it critical to contact emergency services without delay.

Understanding the gravity of these symptoms is just as crucial as recognizing them. Strokes are indeed emergencies just like heart attacks, and they deserve the same level of urgent response. This is a rallying point for empowerment—everyone, regardless of medical background, can take charge in these critical moments by using the FAST protocol.

Remember that strokes are not elder-exclusive events. They can happen to anyone, at any age. Particularly, individuals with heart disease are at an increased risk, but controllable factors like diet, exercise, and stress management can reduce this risk significantly. This knowledge forms a line of defense and gives a sense of control over an individual's health destiny.

Caregivers, as vital links in the chain of support for heart disease patients, should be well versed in the FAST protocol. By staying observant and prepared, they can serve as early responders, ensuring that the crucial window for effective stroke treatment is not missed.

In the context of stroke prevention and response, it's also essential to stay informed about the latest treatments and recovery strategies. The medical community is continuously learning and innovating, with a common goal of preserving life and quality of life. Being current with this knowledge enhances the capacity to advocate for oneself or a loved one in the midst of medical decisions.

For healthcare professionals, the FAST protocol is more than a guide; it embodies the ethical and moral responsibility to educate patients and the public. Empowering people with this information instills a sense of agency that can transform outcomes and improve the overall quality of heart health care.

When faced with a potential stroke, it's crucial to know that there's a system in place for responding quickly and effectively. The FAST protocol is simple, but within its brevity lies the potential to save lives and avert long-term disability. It's a symbol of hope in the face of adversity—a testament to the power of preparedness and immediate action.

Lifestyle modifications, which are extensively detailed in subsequent chapters, form the foundation for reducing the risk of heart disease and stroke. Such changes are testament to one's commitment to heart health and overall well-being. The FAST protocol, however, deals with the more immediate response required in the face of emergent situations, signifying that prevention and preparedness should work hand in hand.

Finally, the FAST protocol supports the broader goal of this book—to educate, motivate, and empower individuals in their heart health journey. It brings together the critical elements of information, response, and intervention that are pivotal during a stroke. This knowledge becomes an integral part of a heart-healthy lifestyle, a piece of wisdom to carry and to share, with the potential to alter fates at a moment's notice.

Let the FAST protocol be understood not just as a response strategy, but as a call to action for those striving for heart health and for those who stand with them. Embrace the knowledge with the confidence that results from an informed and proactive stance on health.

To sum it up, the FAST protocol is a clarion call for immediate action against stroke—a call that reverberates with urgency and necessity. Its principles are simple, its application swift, and its influence wide-reaching. Ingraining this information deep within our collective consciousness can pave the way to a future with fewer strokes and more survivors leading full, vibrant lives.

Chapter 4:
Risk Factors You Can Control

Empowerment begins with understanding the risk factors for heart disease that rest in the palm of your hands, waiting for you to take action. These controllable risks are not mere numbers on a chart; they are lifestyle choices and habits within your sphere of influence. Sustaining a healthy heart extends far beyond the avoidance of smoking; it's a commitment to regulate factors like diabetes and cholesterol through informed dietary decisions and medication adherence when necessary. Recognize that your weight and blood pressure are not arbitrary; they are critical indicators of your heart's health, powerful enough to be manipulated by the strength of your dedication to exercise and nutrition. By taking ownership of these modifiable elements, you craft a shield against heart disease, arming yourself with knowledge and the unwavering resolve to steer your own ship through the turbulent waters towards a place of wellness and vitality.

Smoking and Heart Health

Smoking, an established nemesis of health, stands as one of the most significant modifiable risk factors for heart disease. The combustion of tobacco produces numerous chemicals, each carrying the potential to harm cardiovascular function. Evidently, nicotine and carbon monoxide, to name a couple, play lead roles in this detrimental process. As we delve into the subject of smoking and heart health, we illuminate the intricate ways these substances sabotage the heart's wellbeing, effectively narrowing arteries and reducing the oxygen that reaches the heart muscle.

The mechanics behind smoking's assault on cardiac health are multifaceted. When nicotine invades the bloodstream, it triggers the release of adrenaline, which in turn forces the heart to work harder by increasing heart rate and blood pressure. This repetitive overexertion can eventually lead to chronic hypertension—a silent threat and a precursor to grave cardiac events. Nicotine's other sinister effect includes the stimulation of atherogenesis—the buildup of plaque in the arteries—which impedes the smooth flow of blood.

Carbon monoxide, a byproduct of burnt tobacco, further compounds the problem by binding to hemoglobin more efficiently than oxygen. This dangerous liaison significantly diminishes the oxygen-carrying capacity of the blood, leading to ischemia or lack of oxygen to the heart muscle, which can culminate in a heart attack. Dismally, each puff of a cigarette introduces this harmful gas into the lungs, perpetuating a cycle of oxygen deprivation to vital organs.

Smoking also elicits systemic inflammation, an underlying condition that plays its hand in many chronic diseases, heart disease included. The chemicals in cigarette smoke ignite inflammation within blood vessels, which can lead to the development of arterial plaque. Over time, this inflammatory response can cause the plaque to become unstable, potentially resulting in a full-blown heart attack if the plaque ruptures.

Furthermore, the act of smoking can alter the lipid profile in the blood. It tends to increase the levels of low-density lipoprotein (LDL) cholesterol—often dubbed 'bad cholesterol'—and decrease high-density lipoprotein (HDL) cholesterol, which is protective. This unfavorable shift creates an environment ripe for the progression of coronary artery disease. Consequently, the arteries may harden and narrow, an affliction known as atherosclerosis, which is a leading cause of heart attacks and strokes.

Quitting smoking, therefore, is not a casual recommendation; it is a critical imperative for heart health. Those who relinquish the grip of tobacco can look forward to a slew of health benefits. Within a mere 20 minutes of quitting, blood pressure and heart rate drop to healthier levels. Over the following months and years, the risk of coronary heart disease begins to plummet and can be reduced to that of a non-smoker's in as little as a decade, depending on other health factors.

Thankfully, the cessation of smoking invites an improvement in blood circulation and lung function, allowing for more effective delivery of oxygen to the heart and other organs. This can translate into better exercise tolerance, one of the cornerstones of a heart-healthy lifestyle. Moreover, the reduction in inflammation and the normalization of the lipid profile further tilt the odds in favor of cardiovascular resilience.

The path to becoming smoke-free is not solitary. There are numerous resources available, including nicotine replacement therapies, medications, and behavioral counseling. Each offers a valuable lifeline toward breaking the habitute. A healthcare provider can tailor a quit-smoking plan that aligns with an individual's unique circumstances, enhancing the prospect of success.

For those living with heart disease or at high risk, the significance of smoking cessation cannot be overstated. Each attempt to quit brings one closer to a healthier heart. Rebounding from a relapse, which is common, should be viewed not as failure but as an integral part of the journey toward cessation. Persistence in the face of such challenges embodies the very essence of taking control of one's heart health.

Secondary smoke, too, poses a threat to cardiovascular wellness. Non-smokers who are regularly exposed to smoke can also suffer from the adverse effects on heart health. Hence, creating a smoke-free environment benefits everyone, shielding loved ones from the insidious reach of secondhand smoke's detrimental influence on heart health.

Embarking on this journey may seem daunting, but its reward—a stronger, healthier heart—is a powerful motivator. As you bid farewell to smoking, you'll notice improvements in overall wellness, reinforcing the conviction that this formidable choice is not merely a sacrifice but a reaffirmation of life's value. The heart, after all, is the drumbeat of our existence, and caring for it with such a profound act of self-care is the epitome of empowerment.

Ultimately, the evidence is unequivocal: smoking and heart health are deeply interwoven, and the impact of tobacco on the heart is undeniably destructive. Arming yourself with knowledge, summoning the strength to change, and seeking support are all crucial steps in mitigating this preventable risk factor. The heart's capacity to recover and thrive once liberated from the clutches of tobacco underscores the body's remarkable ability to heal, an assurance that it's never too late to make a change that could literally save your life.

As we move forward in this text, understanding the interface between lifestyle choices and heart health becomes ever more pertinent. Recognizing the monumental benefits of smoking cessation in heart health, we are driven to explore further strategies in subsequent chapters to enhance cardiac function and stave off disease—a pursuit worthy of the heart's vital role in our lives.

Managing Diabetes and Cholesterol

The convergence of diabetes and cholesterol management represents a pivotal axis for protecting your heart health. It's essential to recognize that unmanaged diabetes and high cholesterol levels are not just independent risk factors but often act synergistically, creating a more significant threat to your cardiovascular health. Hence, a clear understanding and proactive management of both conditions are paramount.

Understanding the interplay of these two conditions is critical. Diabetes can impair the body's ability to manage blood sugar levels effectively, and when coupled with dyslipidemia or abnormal cholesterol levels, it magnifies the risk of heart disease. Elevated blood sugar can damage blood vessels and the nerves that control your heart, while high levels of bad cholesterol (LDL) can lead to plaque buildup in arteries, a condition known as atherosclerosis.

To manage diabetes, monitoring your blood glucose levels is essential. Consistent glucose regulation is a cornerstone of diabetes care, achieved through a balanced diet, regular physical activity, and medication if necessary. Your dietary choices can significantly impact your blood glucose and cholesterol levels. Prioritizing foods low in saturated and trans fats, cholesterol, and simple sugars can help manage both diabetes and cholesterol levels.

Maintaining a heart-healthy diet involves consuming plenty of fiber-rich foods such as fruits, vegetables, and whole grains. Soluble fiber, in particular, found in foods like beans, oats, and flaxseed, can aid in lowering LDL cholesterol. These foods can also help regulate blood sugar levels, providing a dual benefit.

When it comes to medication, statins may be prescribed to help lower cholesterol levels. Some individuals with diabetes may need insulin or other diabetes medications to manage their condition. It's imperative to work closely with your healthcare provider to determine the best medication regimen for your specific needs.

Regular physical activity is another pillar in managing both diabetes and cholesterol. Engaging in at least 150 minutes of moderate-intensity aerobic exercise per week is recommended. This can include activities such as brisk walking, cycling, or swimming, which help improve cholesterol levels and aid in glucose control.

It's also important to keep track of your diabetes and cholesterol through regular testing. Hemoglobin A1C tests provide an average blood sugar level over the past two to three months for those with diabetes, while routine blood tests can monitor cholesterol levels. The insight from these tests guides treatment adjustments and lifestyle changes.

Stress management has its role in this symphony of health adjustments. Chronic stress can negatively impact both blood sugar levels and cholesterol, setting the stage for heart disease. Cultivating stress-reducing practices like mindful meditation or deep breathing exercises can support your overall wellness plan.

Moreover, smoking cessation is vital in managing both diabetes and cholesterol. Smoking exacerbates the negative effects of diabetes on your heart and can increase LDL levels while lowering HDL (good) cholesterol, which helps to remove bad cholesterol from your bloodstream.

Weight management is another critical aspect. Carrying excess body weight, particularly around the abdomen, can contribute to insulin resistance and increased LDL cholesterol while decreasing HDL cholesterol. Achieving and maintaining a healthy weight can reduce these risks substantially.

Understanding and being attuned to the medications you take for other conditions is also crucial. Some drugs, including certain diuretics and beta-blockers for high blood pressure, can affect blood glucose and cholesterol levels. This is why coordinating with your healthcare team is indispensable to managing your health holistically.

In your daily life, simple substitutions can make a significant impact. Switching from butter to olive oil, choosing lean proteins, and opting for whole-grain bread over white are small choices that make significant strides in managing cholesterol and diabetes.

Moderation in alcohol consumption is advised, as excessive drinking can lead to an increase in both blood sugar and triglyceride levels, another type of fat in your blood that can increase the risk of heart disease.

Last but not least, the power of community and emotional support can't be overlooked. Joining support groups for individuals with diabetes and heart disease offers a platform to share experiences, tips, and encouragement, which can be key in maintaining the motivation needed for successful long-term management.

A proactive approach to managing diabetes and cholesterol involves regular screenings, lifestyle modifications, medication adherence, and educational empowerment. By taking command of these manageable aspects of your health, you support not just your heart, but also your overall vitality and longevity. You are armed with the knowledge and tools to form robust defenses against heart disease, ensuring your heart continues to thrive and support you through life's journey.

The Importance of Weight and Blood Pressure

As we delve into the crucial aspects of heart health, it's essential to recognize the profound influence of weight and blood pressure on your well-being. These two factors are not merely numbers on a scale or a cuff; they're powerful indicators of your cardiovascular system's condition, and they provide a window into your overall health status.

Understanding the intricate balance within our bodies helps us appreciate the significance of maintaining a healthy weight and optimal blood pressure levels. The excess weight puts undue strain on the heart, demanding more effort for every beat it takes and every movement you make. It's a force that silently but steadily taxes the heart, potentially leading to a host of heart diseases. In the pursuit of heart health, knowledge is power, and action is its faithful companion.

On the other side of the coin, blood pressure tells its own compelling story. Elevated blood pressure, or hypertension, can be likened to the tumultuous waters of a river battering against its banks. When your blood pressure is high, it signifies that your blood is pushing too forcefully against the arterial walls. This relentless force can cause microscopic tears, setting the stage for atherosclerosis—the buildup of plaque, which can lead to catastrophic events like heart attacks and strokes.

Making incremental changes to your diet and physical activity levels can wield significant influence over your weight and blood pressure. Integrating whole, nutrient-dense foods while reducing intake of processed foods high in sodium and unhealthy fats, serves as a stepping stone towards a heart-healthy lifestyle. These therapeutic lifestyle changes can illuminate the path towards not simply living but thriving with vitality.

But beyond diet, the interrelationship between weight and blood pressure extends to other dimensions of our lives. Regular physical activity not only aids in shedding excess weight but also reduces blood pressure, fortifies the heart muscle, and improves blood flow. An active lifestyle is a keystone habit that unlocks numerous cardiovascular benefits.

Monitoring your blood pressure should become as routine as brushing your teeth – it's a daily habit that offers immediate feedback and guides the course of action. Blood pressure monitoring is not just for those diagnosed with hypertension; it's a vigilant measure for everyone conscious of their heart health. When your blood pressure readings begin to rise, it's a signal to take a closer look at lifestyle factors and to consult with healthcare professionals for advice.

Speaking of professional guidance, let's not discount the value of medical support in managing weight and blood pressure. Medications might be necessary, and adherence to prescribed treatments is paramount. But remember that drugs should coexist with – not replace – lifestyle improvements. Their purpose is to complement the foundational changes you're implementing.

Regarding weight management, remember that it's not solely about the digits on the scale. Body composition— the proportion of fat versus muscle—plays a crucial role. Equipping yourself with knowledge about body mass index (BMI) and waist circumference can guide your efforts more accurately. A healthcare professional can help you interpret these measures and suggest personalized strategies for improvement.

It's also worth noting the importance of sleep and its relationship with weight and blood pressure. High-quality sleep renews the heart and the vascular system. A lack of sleep can lead to weight gain and increased blood pressure, destabilizing the heart's rhythm. Prioritizing a good night's sleep is an act of self-care that strengthens the heart.

Don't underestimate the influence of mental and emotional health on your physical condition. Stress can lead to behaviors that contribute to weight gain and elevated blood pressure, such as overeating or inactivity. Cultivating stress management techniques is therefore vital in your heart health regimen.

Amid these discussions, it's important to celebrate every victory along the way. Reward yourself for the pounds shed and the points dropped in blood pressure readings. Acknowledge your progress, for each step forward is a testament to your commitment to heart health.

Understanding genetics is also essential when it comes to weight and blood pressure. Some individuals may be predisposed to certain conditions, but that doesn't render them powerless. Genetics may load the gun, but lifestyle pulls the trigger. You can influence your destiny through the choices you make daily.

Finally, in the expansive journey of heart health, weight and blood pressure are critical landmarks. They inform us about our current state and inspire actions to move toward optimal health. With a proactive attitude, each of us holds the power to shape our heart health destiny, one choice, and one day at a time.

Embrace these metrics as your allies in the quest for a robust heart. See them not as rigid numbers that define you but as dynamic figures that guide you. Let them be the compass that steers you towards healthier habits, a fuller life, and a future where your heart beats strong. Take charge today, for your heart is the drumbeat to the rhythm of your life.

Chapter 5:
Risk Factors You Cannot Control

In the realm of heart health, not all risk factors bow to our will; some are etched in the bedrock of our being, beyond the reach of even the most steadfast efforts. Acknowledge the genes that whisper the history of your forebears, for they carry tales of heart health that may affect your own narrative. Embrace the natural progression of life, too, as age weaves its inevitable silver threads into your story, and recognize that, particularly for women, the transformative phase of menopause marks not just a change in life, but a shift in cardiac risk. Understanding these elements, which spell your unique susceptibility to cardiovascular disease, is not about surrender but about awareness. It's a pivot from feeling powerless in the face of unmodifiable risk factors to adopting a determined stance where knowledge fuels vigilance and propels you towards meticulous monitoring—a journey underpinned by empowerment and prudent, preventive care.

Genetics and Family History

As we continue to explore heart health and endeavor to understand the myriad factors influencing its condition, we must turn our attention to the complex and intriguing role that genetics and family history play in the context of heart disease. These ingrained elements, often beyond our immediate control, establish a framework within which our personal health narrative is written. But while they may set the stage, remember that they do not dictate the final act. There is profound power in understanding these aspects, and interactive steps can be taken to mitigate their impact.

The intricate blueprint of our DNA holds key information about our susceptibility to various conditions, including heart disease. Certain genetic markers and variations can predispose us to elevated risks of heart disease, even with a seemingly optimal lifestyle in place. The heritability of heart disease is significant – if your immediate family members have a history of heart-related issues, it's crucial to take that history seriously.

Heart disease can cluster in families due to genetic factors, shared environment, or a combination of both. Family traits such as high blood pressure, cholesterol levels, and tendencies towards diabetes are often passed down the generations, creating a familial pattern that can be observed and anticipated. These patterns, while indicative of risk, do not necessarily seal one's fate; they serve as red flags signaling the need for heightened awareness and proactive behavior.

Understanding the genetic nuances of heart disease is an evolving science. Research has identified specific genes associated with increased risk for heart conditions like arrhythmias, congenital heart defects, and cardiomyopathies. Genetic testing is an area growing in sophistication, offering individuals insight into their personal risk factors. However, it is paramount to approach genetic testing with expert guidance, ensuring the results are interpreted with care and appropriate context.

Inherited conditions such as familial hypercholesterolemia cause very high levels of cholesterol and can significantly increase the risk of heart disease at an early age. Such conditions warrant vigilant monitoring and management, emphasizing the necessity of informed medical partnerships and consistent health check-ups.

One's gender plays a fundamental role in how genetics affect heart disease risk. Women, for instance, may experience unique genetic predispositions that interplay with factors such as hormonal changes during menopause. Understanding these gender-specific genetic influinfluences can refine prevention strategies and personalize care.

While you can't change your genetic make-up, knowing your family history empowers you to speak with healthcare providers about your own risks for heart disease. This conversation has the potential to inform decisions about lifestyle adjustments and necessary medical interventions that can safeguard your heart's health.

Lifestyle factors such as diet, exercise, and stress management demonstrate an ability to modify the expression of genes, a promising field known as epigenetics. Therefore, even with a family history of heart disease, adopting and maintaining heart-healthy habits is doubly important. These actions can potentially dampen the effect of genetic predispositions and pave the way for a stronger, healthier heart.

Genetic considerations also extend to pharmacogenomics – the study of how someone's genetic make-up affects their response to drugs. Recognizing the genetic aspects of heart disease can guide health professionals in personalizing medication regimens that are most effective and least likely to cause side effects for each individual.

Pregnancy-related complications such as eclampsia or gestational diabetes can signal an increased risk for cardiovascular disease later in life, revealing yet another facet of how family history, particularly maternal health, is entwined with heart disease risk. Women need to be aware of these risks, not only for themselves but for the health literacy of their families.

Knowing your family's heart health history isn't simply about awareness. It should inspire action. Take this knowledge to your healthcare providers, discuss screening options, and consider regular monitoring for heart health indicators such as blood pressure, cholesterol, and glucose levels. Make genetic and family history part of your ongoing dialogue about your health.

Finally, reach out to your relatives to understand their health status as part of building your family's health history. Such conversations, while perhaps delicate, are vital. Shared knowledge among family members can foster collective preventive measures and support networks that benefit everyone involved.

Encouragingly, your genetic and familial predispositions need not be a source of anxiety but rather a catalyst for empowerment and informed action. With the right approach, the data points of your lineage transform from a forecast to a roadmap – a guide towards a heart-smart lifestyle tailored to your unique genetic identity.

To encapsulate, genetics and family history are undeniable contributors to the risk of heart disease, yet they represent starting points for intervention rather than deterministic endpoints. With conscientious care, targeted prevention, and lifestyle optimization, you can author a more promising heart health story for yourself, regardless of the script genetics has provided.

Let's embrace our genetic heritage not as a destiny but as a call to action. An awareness of your family history dovetailed with a proactive stance on health can create a buffer against genetic predispositions. Your heart's future can be resilient – informed by your past, but not restricted by it. The steps you take today resonate far beyond yourself, potentially altering the health legacy you pass down to future generations. Therein lies an inspiring opportunity to redefine the narrative of heart health within the tapestry of genetics and family history.

Age and Menopause Considerations

When embarking on the journey of understanding heart health, particularly in women, it's crucial to recognize the roles age and menopause play. The fluctuating landscape of female hormones throughout a woman's life can markedly influence heart disease risk. In the spirit of strengthening your heart's resilience, this section dives into age-related changes and the intersection of menopause, providing a deeper understanding and actionable insights to support your heart.

As we age, our bodies undergo a myriad of changes, and the heart is no exception. With each passing year, the heart must adapt to the evolving demands and alterations within the circulatory system. This can manifest as a natural stiffening of the blood vessels and heart muscles, making it more challenging for the heart to pump with the same vigor it once did. Such changes necessitate a heightened focus on maintaining cardiovascular health, especially as one approaches midlife.

For women, menopause marks a significant transition, one where the protective effects of estrogen are reduced. Estrogen is believed to have a beneficial impact on the inner layer of artery walls, assisting in keeping blood vessels flexible. Therefore, as estrogen levels decline, women may see an uptick in risk factors associated with cardiovascular diseases. Understanding this shift is key to preemptive heart care.

It's imperative to consider that heart disease doesn't happen overnight. Risk factors accumulate over the years, evolving silently. During the premenopausal years, women can take preemptive strikes against heart disease by focusing on a healthy lifestyle. This includes a balanced diet, regular exercise, and managing blood pressure and cholesterol levels—practices that build a solid foundation for heart health as one ages.

When women enter perimenopause, often in their 40s and 50s, they may begin to experience changes in their cardiovascular health. Blood pressure and cholesterol levels may start to rise. It's not uncommon for weight gain to occur during this time as well, potentially leading to increased abdominal fat—a known risk factor for heart disease.

As the menopausal transition progresses, the risk of developing heart-related issues can increase. Symptoms like hot flashes and night sweats are well-documented, but it's equally important to be vigilant about heart palpitations, changes in lipid profiles, and increased blood pressure. Monitoring these changes and discussing them with a healthcare professional can be crucial in minimizing their impact on heart health.

Lifestyle interventions become even more critical as menopause approaches. A heart-healthy diet rich in fruits, vegetables, whole grains, lean proteins, and healthy fats supports cardiovascular health. Regular physical activity, including both aerobic and resistance exercises, helps maintain a healthy weight and strengthens the heart muscles.

Postmenopausal women have a higher incidence of cardiovascular diseases compared to their younger counterparts—an indisputable reason for prioritizing heart health screenings. After menopause, screenings should become more frequent, with a focus on tracking blood pressure, cholesterol, blood sugar, and body mass index (BMI). These metrics provide invaluable insights into your cardiovascular well-being.

While lifestyle modifications are powerful, hormone replacement therapy (HRT) is a topic often broached in conversations about managing menopausal symptoms. It's essential to understand the potential benefits and risks associated with HRT and how it may impact your heart. Decisions regarding HRT should be made with careful consideration and consultation with a healthcare provider who understands your unique cardiovascular risk profile.

Managing stress during these years cannot be overstated in its importance for heart health. Stress can exacerbate menopause symptoms and has a direct impact on blood pressure and heart rate. Developing coping strategies like deep breathing, meditation, yoga, or other relaxation techniques is not just about inner calm—it's a fortification for your heart.

Don't underestimate the power of sleep. As hormone levels fluctuate, sleep may become elusive for many women, yet restorative sleep is a pillar of heart health. It is during deep sleep that your heart rate slows, blood pressure drops, and the heart has a chance to recover from the day's demands. Prioritizing sleep hygiene practices ensures that your heart gets the rest it needs.

Another critical consideration for aging women is calcium and vitamin D intake to support bone health. However, it's important to balance bone health with cardiovascular health, as excessive calcium can contribute to heart disease. Tailoring your intake to your specific needs, while keeping an eye on your heart, is a delicate yet manageable balance.

Finally, a word about the significance of community and support networks during this time of transition. Emotional support from friends, families, and support groups can provide solace and encouragement. Sharing experiences, concerns, and successes with others fosters a sense of empowerment and can have a heartwarming effect on your overall well-being.

Through all these considerations, it's paramount to remain proactive rather than reactive about heart health. Menopause is a natural stage of life, one that can be met with awareness and thoughtful care. By taking control of the risk factors that can be influenced, and by working in collaboration with healthcare providers, women can navigate this period with strength and minimize their risk of heart disease. Embrace this time as an opportunity to renew your commitment to a heart-healthy lifestyle and let the wisdom of age be your guide.

In conclusion, age and menopause are landmarks in a woman's life that can bring about various heart health challenges. Yet these same challenges hold the potential to transform your health journey. With each proactive step, you bolster your heart's defenses and enrich your life. Awareness, vigilance, and intentional action are the cornerstones of this transformation, and with them, you have the power to forge a heart-resilient future.

Chapter 6:
The Heart-Smart Diet

Emerging seamlessly from the shadows of uncontrollable risk factors, Chapter 6 shifts our focus to the transformative power of dietary choices in bolstering heart health. The Heart-Smart Diet isn't a fleeting trend; it's a sustainable pathway towards nurturing your heart with every bite. This chapter unveils the foundational principles of a diet that sings in harmony with your heart's needs. You'll learn to discern between villainous fats that lurk in the guise of comfort foods and the heroic unsaturated fats that stand as your heart's allies. We'll untangle the complexities of sugars and spotlight nutrient-dense champions that not only empower your palate but also energize your cardiovascular system. This journey through the heart-smart diet is designed to leave you feeling informed, inspired, and invigorated, ready to embrace the delectable delights of foods that work tirelessly for your ticker's triumph.

Essentials of a Heart-Healthy Diet

Embracing a heart-healthy diet is pivotal in the pursuit of improving cardiovascular well-being and minimizing the risks associated with heart disease. The choices one makes in the kitchen can significantly influence the health of one's heart and overall vitality.

The cornerstone of a heart-healthy diet is diversity—integrating a colorful array of foods rich in nutrients that are vital for maintaining a robust heart. Fruits and vegetables, with their high content of essential vitamins, minerals, and fiber, should be the bedrock of such a diet. Eating a variety of these plant-based foods not only supports heart function but also contributes to overall health.

Whole grains are another essential component. Foods like brown rice, quinoa, oats, and whole wheat are packed with fiber which can help maintain a healthy weight and reduce cholesterol levels — a crucial factor in preventing heart disease. Integrating whole grains into one's diet can be both delicious and beneficial for one's heart.

Lean proteins such as poultry, fish, and plant-based alternatives are vital for a balanced diet that supports heart health. Fish rich in omega-3 fatty acids, such as salmon, tuna, and mackerel, are particularly beneficial for the heart, as they help reduce inflammation and lower the risk of rhythm disorders.

Moreover, legumes like beans, lentils, and chickpeas are nutritious powerhouses that provide protein without the saturated fat found in some animal proteins. They are an excellent choice for anyone looking to improve their heart's health while still enjoying fulfilling meals.

The role of healthy fats cannot be overstated. One should aim for unsaturated fats found in olive oil, avocados, and nuts, which can help reduce the levels of harmful LDL cholesterol and raise beneficial HDL cholesterol. This balance is instrumental in preventing plaque buildup in arteries.

Portion control is another key aspect. Eating in moderation ensures you get a sufficient amount of nutrients without overloading your system with unnecessary calories. This can help maintain a healthy weight, which significantly impacts blood pressure, cholesterol levels, and the risk of heart disease.

Hydration is also critical. Consuming an ample amount of water daily supports every function in your body, including heart rate and blood pressure. Limiting intake of beverages high in sugars and caffeine can help maintain heart rhythm and pressure.

Reducing sodium intake is essential for heart health. High sodium levels can lead to hypertension, a leading cause of heart disease. Cooking fresh meals at home allows you to control the amount of sodium, as opposed to consuming processed foods that are typically high in salt.

It's also crucial to limit the intake of added sugars found in many processed foods and sweetened beverages. High sugar consumption can lead to obesity, inflammation, high blood pressure, and diabetes—all risk factors for heart disease.

Consistency in maintaining a heart-healthy diet is essential but so is flexibility. Allowing oneself the occasional indulgence is not only psychologically rewarding but can also help you maintain a long-term healthy eating pattern without feeling deprived.

Beyond individual foods, building a heart-healthy plate is about combining these essentials in balance. Half of the plate should be filled with fruits and vegetables, a quarter with whole grains, and the remaining quarter with lean proteins, complemented by a modest amount of healthy fats.

Lastly, developing and maintaining habits such as reading food labels, cooking at home, and mindful eating can have a transformative impact on one's heart health. Understanding the nutritional content of your food and being present with each bite encourages healthier food choices and portion sizes.

The path to a healthy heart is paved with small, daily decisions. By making intentional, informed choices about the foods we consume, we forge a strong defense against heart disease and stride confidently towards health and longevity.

Remember, the power to shape your heart health is on your plate. With every meal, you have the opportunity to nourish your heart and honor the body that serves you. Embrace the journey of creating a heart-healthy diet as an act of self-respect and a commitment to a vibrant, empowered life.

Understanding Fats and Sugars

Diving deeper into the heart-smart diet, one critical aspect which often garners both confusion and concern is the role of fats and sugars. These macronutrients are energy sources, but they differ vastly in their impact on cardiovascular health. A nuanced understanding of fats and sugars is essential for managing heart disease effectively.

Fats are not the enemy of heart health as was once widely believed. In fact, certain fats play a vital role in maintaining bodily functions and are necessary for good health. Unsaturated fats, which include polyunsaturated and monounsaturated fats, are known to be heart-healthy as they can help reduce bad cholesterol levels and lower the risk of heart disease and stroke when they replace saturated fats in the diet.

On the other hand, saturated fats found in red meat, full-fat dairy products, and trans fats, often lurking in processed and fried foods, can increase blood cholesterol levels and plaque formation in arteries. Here, moderation is key. While it's not practical to eliminate these entirely, as they often come packaged with beneficial nutrients, their limited consumption is imperative.

An important dietary shift is the reduction of trans fats, which are the most detrimental to heart health. Trans fats not only increase bad cholesterol (LDL) but also lower good cholesterol (HDL), doubling the risk to heart health. Fortunately, awareness and food regulations have reduced their presence in our diets, but vigilance remains necessary.

With sugars, the message is clearer: excessive intake is harmful to heart health. Added sugars contribute to obesity, inflammation, high cholesterol, and diabetes—all risk factors for heart disease. Moreover, sugars do not possess any essential nutrients, which makes them empty calories, providing energy with no nutritional benefit.

Natural sugars, found in fruits, vegetables, and dairy, are part of a healthy diet, but even these should be consumed thoughtfully, especially in the context of other health concerns like diabetes. The real issue lies with added sugars in sodas, baked goods, and even savory foods where they lurk unnoticed. The recommendation to not exceed more than 10% of daily calories from added sugars is a guideline motivated by substantial evidence.

For individuals with heart disease, cutting back on added sugars is a strategic move towards better health outcomes. Replacing sugary beverages with water or unsweetened drinks, enjoying fruit instead of dessert, and carefully reading food labels to avoid hidden sugars can make significant improvements in dietary patterns.

Another angle to consider is the glycemic index of foods. Foods high in added sugars often have a high glycemic index, causing spikes in blood glucose levels. These spikes can over time lead to insulin resistance, a precursor to type 2 diabetes, which is a significant risk factor for heart disease.

It's also useful to understand the interplay between fats and sugars. Sometimes, low-fat products increase added sugars to compensate for loss in flavor, which can be counterproductive for individuals trying to improve their heart health. Balancing fats and sugars for an overall heart-healthy diet involves recognizing these trade-offs and making informed choices.

But beyond the physiological impact, it's imperative to integrate this knowledge into a livable, enjoyable dietary pattern. This change is about finding harmony in nourishment rather than strict avoidance, focusing on nutrient-dense, fiber-rich foods that satisfy and support heart health.

A steadfast ally in this dietary transformation is the nutrition label. Learning to decipher nutritional facts not only empowers you to make better choices but also encourages mindfulness about what enters your body, facilitating a direct connection between nutrition and its effects on the heart.

Understand, too, that this knowledge is not a call to perfection but rather an encouragement to make more heart-conscious choices daily. Improvement is a process; each step towards reducing fats and sugars in favor of more wholesome options is a victory for your heart.

Embrace the complexity of nutrients and engage with your food choices with curiosity and flexibility. Explore the myriad of alternatives available—substitute saturated fats with healthier fats like olive oil, enjoy a lush avocado instead of butter, and let natural sweetness from fruits replace the usual spoonful of sugar.

In conclusion, understanding fats and sugars in the context of heart health isn't about demonizing these macronutrients but about informing yourself to make knowledgeable decisions that align with your health goals. It's about creating a diet that's as good for your taste buds as it is for your heart. And above all, it's about taking control and realizing that with each mindful meal, you're not just eating; you're nurturing the very core of your vitality—your heart.

Heart-Boosting Foods and Nutrients

Moving forward in our exploration of heart health, let's delve into the empowering choices you can make right in your kitchen. Our diet plays a monumental role in heart health, providing the building blocks our hearts need to stay strong and resilient. Here, we'll focus on the specific foods and nutrients that can have a positive impact on your heart's well-being. Taking the reins of your diet can be transformative, enriching your body with heart-boosting essentials.

Firstly, let's consider the critical role of omega-3 fatty acids. Found abundantly in oily fish such as salmon, mackerel, and sardines, these polyunsaturated fats are central to reducing inflammation, one of the key players in heart disease. Including fish in your diet a couple of times a week, or supplementing with fish oil, can support heart rhythm and reduce the risk of heart attack and stroke.

When it comes to omega-3s, it's not only fish that can bolster your heart health. Flaxseeds and chia seeds are plant sources rich in alpha-linolenic acid (ALA), a type of omega-3 fatty acid. Integrating ground seeds into your meals or smoothies can be an easy and effective way to enhance your omega-3 intake.

Antioxidants are another ally in the fight against heart disease. Foods that boast a high antioxidant content, such as berries, dark leafy greens, and dark chocolate, can help mitigate oxidative stress which impacts the health of your blood vessels. These wholesome foods can be savored as sweet treats or hearty salads – flexible options for any meal plan.

Whole grains hold an integral spot on our list of heart-boosting foods. By choosing whole grains over refined grains, you're embracing a source of soluble fiber, which is known to help lower cholesterol levels. Oats, brown rice, and quinoa are more than just side dishes; they're supporters enlisted in maintaining your heart's rhythm and health.

Magnesium is a mineral to note for its heart-helping properties. Present in foods such as nuts, seeds, legumes, and leafy greens, magnesium aids in regulating blood pressure, a crucial factor for preventing heart strain. An approach as simple as snacking on a handful of almonds or preparing a spinach-based meal can significantly contribute to your heart's magnesium needs.

Don't overlook the importance of potassium; this mineral helps maintain electrical gradients in your cells and manages blood pressure levels. Bananas, oranges, sweet potatoes, and tomatoes are convenient, potassium-packed choices that fit seamlessly into a heart-conscious diet.

Nuts and seeds deserve their own highlight. Not only are they sources of omega-3 and magnesium, but they also contain mono- and polyunsaturated fats, which can help lower bad cholesterol levels when consumed in moderation. They're a snack that serves a purpose beyond mere satisfaction; they're little guardians of your heart's health.

Vegetables such as carrots, spinach, and broccoli are not just about adding color to your plate; these are high in fiber and vitamins which play a part in reducing the risk of coronary heart disease. Embrace these nutritional powerhouses by experimenting with creative ways of cooking that preserve their heart-protective nutrients.

As we look beyond singular foods, let's not forget the potency of compound effects. A heart-healthy diet is often characterized by the Mediterranean diet, which emphasizes fruits, vegetables, whole grains, and healthy fats. By taking cues from this diet, you can synergistically combine the diverse array of heart-boosting foods and maximize their benefits for your cardiovascular system.

Limiting sodium is another tactic you can employ to protect your heart. Instead of reaching for the salt shaker, try enhancing your meals with spices, herbs, and citrus to reduce your risk of high blood pressure and heart disease. This strategy isn't about sacrificing flavor but rather discovering new taste profiles that benefit your heart.

Let's talk about the beverages that keep you hydrated and your heart content. Green tea is celebrated for its catechins and flavonoids, antioxidant compounds that can improve blood vessel function and decrease inflammation. So next time you're choosing a drink, consider the heart-boosting potential steeped within a cup of green tea.

Also, the power of water should never be underestimated. Staying well-hydrated helps your heart pump blood more easily and maintains the balance of electrolytes essential for heart function. It's a simple yet effective way to support your cardiovascular system throughout the day.

Finally, harness the sweetness of fruits in moderation. While fruits do contain natural sugars, they are also rich in essential nutrients and fiber that help counteract the potential negative effects of sugar. Opting for a piece of fruit rather than a sugar-laden snack is a wise choice that aligns with a heart-smart dietary pattern.

When approaching the realm of heart-boosting foods and nutrients, remember that no single food holds the key to heart health, but rather it is the sum of your daily choices that creates the most impact. By focusing on a diverse and balanced diet with the foods mentioned, you are taking proactive steps to nourish and defend one of your body's most vital organs. Let your heart reap the rewards of your conscious nutritional selections, and allow this knowledge to be a source of encouragement as you build a lifestyle that promotes optimal heart health.

Chapter 7:
Fitness for a Strong Heart

Turning the page from nutrition to physical activity, Chapter 7 delves into the cornerstone of cardiovascular vitality: exercise. Your heart—this indefatigable muscle—thrives on movement. It's vital to understand how to calibrate your fitness regimen for maximum cardiac benefit, and this chapter will serve as your compass. Embarking on a fitness journey need not be daunting; every stride, stretch, and strength exercise is a love letter to your heart. We'll explore how to craft a workout program that aligns with your unique life circumstances, ensuring that it's not just effective, but also sustainable and enjoyable. Whether you're taking your first steps towards fitness or looking to elevate an existing routine, the marriage of cardiovascular and strength training we propose is tailored to fortify your heart, enhance your endurance, and uplift your spirit. Remember, each heartbeat fueled by your dedication to fitness is a testament to your devotion to health. So let's step confidently towards forging a powerful shield for your most precious organ—your strong heart.

Creating Your Heart-Healthy Exercise Routine

As we delve into the essence of heart health, it becomes clear that building a dedicated exercise routine is vital. We're not just striving for longevity; we're aiming for a robust heart, for vitality that permeates every aspect of our lives. Exercise has a profound ability to fortify our hearts, and establishing a heart-healthy routine can be both life-changing and life-saving.

The journey starts with understanding the distinction between physical activity and structured exercise. Both are beneficial, yet it's the routine of regular, structured exercise that yields consistent, measurable improvements to heart health. Your exercise routine should be tailored to your current state of health, taking into account any physical limitations and aligning with your goals for heart wellness.

First, have a conversation with your healthcare provider. It's essential to evaluate your current cardiovascular health status and clarify any restrictions you might have. This is especially important if you have a history of heart disease or are currently starting an exercise routine for the first time after a diagnosis. Once you have the green light, the next step is to devise a plan that matches your individual needs.

Begin with setting clear, achievable goals. If your daily life has been mostly sedentary, a goal might be as simple as incorporating a ten-minute walk into your routine three times a week and gradually increasing the duration and frequency. It's not just about getting moving; it's about building a sustainable habit that your heart can rely on for years to come.

An ideal heart-healthy exercise regimen involves a blend of cardiovascular, strength training, and flexibility exercises. Aerobic activities like walking, jogging, swimming, or cycling are excellent for improving the efficiency of your cardiovascular system. They encourage heart rate elevation and promote increased blood flow, which over time can lower the risk of heart events.

Strength training, done a few times a week, complements your cardio routine by building muscle mass and supporting metabolic health. While lifting weights, using resistance bands, or engaging in bodyweight exercises like squats and push-ups, you're helping your heart in more subtle, equally significant ways.

Don't overlook flexibility and balance exercises. Practices like yoga and tai chi not only improve flexibility but also contribute to a mind-body connection that can reduce stress—a known risk factor for heart disease. These activities can also improve the ability to perform daily activities, which in turn keeps you more active overall.

One of the keys to success is regularity. Your heart thrives on consistency, so strive to exercise at the same time every day to help establish a powerful habit. Whether it's morning, afternoon, or evening, find a window that aligns with your natural rhythms and preferences to ensure better adherence to your routine.

It's also important to track your progress. Monitoring how often you exercise, your session lengths, and the intensity helps in gauging improvements. Use a journal or smartphone app; you'll want a tangible record of your journey that can motivate you during times when progress seems to wane.

When it comes to intensity, be mindful of starting slow. Particularly for individuals with heart disease, it is crucial to incrementally increase the intensity of workouts to avoid overburdening the heart. Low to moderate intensity is often recommended initially, with gradual adjustments made as endurance and strength improve.

Variation in your workout routine can prevent boredom and muscle overuse. Alter your activities, change the scenery, and switch things up to keep both your mind and body engaged. This can help sustain long-term commitment and prevent hitting a plateau in your heart health journey.

Listen to your body's cues. While pushing through a tough workout can sometimes lead to breakthroughs, distinguishing between good pain and harmful discomfort is crucial. Any signs of chest pain, undue breathlessness, or undue fatigue warrant immediate rest and consultation with your healthcare provider.

Combining exercise with other lifestyle changes enhances the heart benefits. A healthy diet, proper sleep, stress reduction, and avoiding harmful substances like tobacco and excessive alcohol should complement your exercise regime. All these components work synergistically to amplify your heart health.

Finally, find a support system. Exercise partners, online communities, or local clubs can provide camaraderie and accountability, two powerful forces in sustaining a heart-healthy exercise regime. Encouragement from friends, family, or like-minded individuals on similar journeys can make all the difference.

Your heart-healthy exercise routine is more than a checklist; it's a commitment to your heart's future and a declaration that your health is a priority. It's not just about the exercise—it's about cultivating an environment that continuously nurtures and supports the heart. As you breathe through each step or lift, you're not just becoming stronger; you're actively participating in a life-affirming process—one that cherishes and celebrates every beat of your heart.

The Benefits of Cardiovascular and Strength Training

As we journey towards better heart health, let's delve into two key components of a heart-healthy exercise routine: cardiovascular and strength training. Both elements offer vast benefits that, when combined, provide a formidable defense against heart disease and empower our overall health and vitality. It's critical to acknowledge that the heart is not just an organ that pumps blood—it's a muscle, and like any muscle in the body, it needs regular exercise to stay strong and efficient.

Engaging in cardiovascular exercise is akin to giving your heart a workout. When we perform activities such as brisk walking, cycling, or swimming, our heart rate increases, bolstering the heart's pumping capacity and improving cardiac output. Embracing such activities for at least 150 minutes a week can significantly reduce the risk of developing heart disease, control weight, and lower blood pressure. But the benefits extend beyond the heart—cardiovascular training enhances lung capacity, increases energy levels, reduces stress, and can even elevate your mood through the release of endorphins.

Strength training, often overshadowed by its cardiovascular counterpart, is equally essential for a heart-healthy lifestyle. Incorporating resistance exercises like weight lifting, Pilates, or body-weight movements can improve muscular strength and endurance. This, in turn, promotes better metabolism which can help with weight management—a critical factor in heart disease prevention. Furthermore, strength training helps combat the loss of muscle mass associated with aging, keeping you agile and independent as you age.

When combined, cardiovascular and strength training create a synergy that maximizes heart health benefits. Strength training can contribute to a healthier body composition by increasing muscle mass, which in turn can improve insulin sensitivity and result in better blood sugar control—a boon for those managing diabetes, a significant heart disease risk factor. Meanwhile, cardiovascular exercise continues to improve heart and lung function, providing a comprehensive exercise plan that addresses several risk factors simultaneously.

Another advantage of incorporating both training methods is the reduction of arterial stiffness—a condition that can lead to hypertension and cardiovascular events. Flexing our muscles against resistance can improve arterial flexibility, allowing blood to flow more freely and reducing strain on the heart. Moreover, by lowering body fat, we can also reduce inflammation within the body, which plays a prominent role in plaque build-up in the arteries.

Strength training should be approached with caution and proper technique to maximize benefits and minimize injury risk, especially for individuals with pre-existing heart conditions. It's vital to start slowly, focusing on light weights and higher repetitions before gradually increasing intensity. Always consult with healthcare professionals or a certified fitness expert to tailor a safe and effective strength training regimen specific to your health needs.

It is also worth noting that cardiovascular exercise doesn't only have to be long sessions at the gym on a treadmill or an elliptical machine. Daily activities that increase the heart rate, such as taking the stairs instead of the elevator, gardening, or even energetic housecleaning, can contribute to your cardiovascular health. The key is consistency and integrating these activities into your daily routine for sustained heart health.

Moreover, practicing strength training can lead to improved bone density, an essential factor for preventing osteoporosis—a concern particularly for women as they age. This enhanced bone strength also means a reduced risk of fractures, which can significantly influence quality of life and autonomy.

For those concerned about gaining excessive bulk from strength training, rest assured that building large muscles requires significant, specialized effort beyond standard strength exercises. Instead, routine strength training will help you achieve a toned and lean physique, and the metabolic boost from increased muscle mass will make it easier to maintain a healthy weight.

Don't forget that exercise also holds incredible psychological benefits. The empowerment that comes from feeling stronger and more capable cannot be overstated, and the improved self-esteem is a significant factor in adhering to a heart-healthy lifestyle. Furthermore, regular physical activity has been shown to alleviate symptoms of depression and anxiety, conditions that can acutely impact heart health.

One of the most profound benefits of cardiovascular and strength training is their impact on longevity and the quality of that extended life. By reducing the risk of chronic conditions associated with heart disease and promoting a robust and resilient body, these exercises enable us to lead active, fulfilling lives well into our later years.

Committing to a blend of cardiovascular and strength training can also improve sleep quality, another crucial element of heart health. Regular physical exertion can help regulate circadian rhythms, leading to more restorative sleep, which provides the body with time to repair and rejuvenate itself.

The societal benefits shouldn't be overlooked either. Adopting these healthy behaviors sets a positive example for our communities, encouraging others to prioritize their heart health. Since heart disease remains the leading cause of death worldwide, fostering a culture of prevention through exercise can have a profound impact on public health.

Lastly, engaging in regular physical activity, including cardiovascular and strength training, fosters a sense of control over one's own health. In a world where so much can feel uncertain, taking proactive steps to strengthen your heart and body is an act of self-care and an investment in your future.

Remember, it's never too late to start. Whether you're already living with heart disease or you're looking to prevent it, incorporating cardiovascular and strength training into your routine can ignite transformative effects on your heart health. With each step taken, each weight lifted, you are building not just muscle, but resilience, determination, and a heart fortified to beat strongly for years to come.

In conclusion, cardiovascular and strength training are twin pillars of heart health, each supporting and reinforcing the benefits of the other. Their combined force offers a powerful means to combat heart disease and elevate your overall well-being. Start where you are, use what you have, do what you can, and watch as your heart responds with vigor and vitality.

Chapter 8:
Stress, Mental Health, and Your Heart

Embarking further into our heart health odyssey, let's pivot toward a less discussed yet crucial pillar of well-being: the dynamic trio of stress, mental health, and your heart. Scripted by life's inevitable challenges, stress scripts a silent saga of cardiovascular strain. It's a clandestine culprit cloaking itself in everyday turmoil but wield a mighty impact on heart health. Yet, recognition can empower resilience. Within this expanse of self-discovery, we integrate practices that not only buffer the heart against the serrated edges of stress but also foster an oasis of mental peace. Embrace strategies that intertwine mindfulness with a robust heart, guiding you to a realm where your pulse beats in harmony with a tranquil mind. As we delve into the nuanced interplay between emotional turbulence and arterial vitality, remember: mastering the art of inner calm isn't just an act of self-care; it's a lifeline to your heart's enduring rhythm.

The Connection Between Stress and Heart Disease

Understanding the intertwining pathways of stress and heart disease is crucial in the quest for optimal heart health. While many physical factors contribute to cardiovascular disease, we cannot underestimate the impact that our mental and emotional well-being has on our heart. This section delves into the intricate relationship between everyday stressors and the health of our most vital organ.

The notion that stress can have real, physiological effects on the heart is supported by numerous studies. These investigations reveal how stress triggers a cascade of hormonal responses, including the release of adrenaline and cortisol. These "stress hormones" ready the body for the "fight or flight" response, which in the short term is protective, but when activated too frequently or for too long, can have damaging repercussions on cardiovascular health.

It's instructive to consider exactly how these stress hormones impact the heart. When released into the bloodstream, they elevate heart rate and blood pressure, temporarily increasing the heart's workload. In a moment of acute stress, these changes are entirely appropriate, but chronic stress keeps the body in a constant state of high alert, which can lead to hypertension—a major risk factor for heart disease.

Beyond blood pressure and heart rate, stress affects the body in other ways that have implications for heart health. For instance, chronic stress has been associated with inflammation, which is a recognized component of atherosclerotic plaque formation. These plaques are the culprit behind many forms of heart disease, as they can limit or block blood flow to vital organs, including the heart itself, leading to conditions such as coronary artery disease.

The close association between stress and behavior is another link in the stress-heart disease chain. When under stress, many individuals are more likely to engage in unhealthy behaviors such as smoking, excessive drinking, and overeating. Each of these behaviors can exacerbate risk factors for heart disease, creating a compoundingly negative effect on heart health.

Furthermore, the impact of emotional stress, particularly conditions such as depression and anxiety, also translates to increased cardiovascular risk. These emotional states can engender a sense of fatigue or demotivation, often leading individuals to forego exercise and other heart-healthy activities. Links have also been found between depression and altered blood clotting, which could increase the risk of heart attack.

Another stress-related condition that deserves attention is the "broken heart syndrome," also known as stress cardiomyopathy. This condition mimics the symptoms of a heart attack and is often triggered by acute emotional stress. While patients typically recover with proper care, it underscores the potency of emotional stress on heart function.

Moving to a more positive note, it's empowering to recognize that stress is manageable. Techniques such as mindfulness, deep breathing exercises, and yoga can mitigate the body's stress response, leading to potential cardiovascular benefits. Adopting these practices into your lifestyle can not only improve your general well-being but can also directly support heart health.

Adapting to stress is also about perception and attitude. Reframing stressful situations into challenges that can be met and mastered, rather than threats that are overwhelming, can significantly modify the stress response. Such reframing can be developed through cognitive behavioral therapy and other psychoeducational interventions.

Incorporating regular physical activity is an excellent way to combat stress and its effects on the heart. Exercise releases endorphins, which can alleviate stress and mood symptoms, and also helps to maintain weight, lower blood pressure, and improve cholesterol levels—all potential contributors to heart health.

Nutrition plays a significant role as well. A diet rich in fruits, vegetables, lean proteins, and whole grains can provide the necessary nutrients to bolster the body's defenses against the impacts of stress, while also reducing inflammation and improving overall heart function.

Additionally, strong social support networks have been recognized as a buffer against stress. Maintaining relationships with friends, family, and supportive communities can provide emotional solace and advice, often helping to lighten the load of stressors faced on a daily basis.

Sleep must not be overlooked either. Adequate sleep is a pillar of stress management and heart health. During sleep, the body works to repair itself, consolidating memories, and reducing the levels of stress hormones. Poor sleep can exacerbate stress, create mood disturbances, and contribute negatively to heart health.

Finally, regular follow-ups with healthcare professionals can ensure that stress-related impacts on heart health are identified early and managed effectively. Your healthcare provider can suggest strategies specific to your situation, which may include pharmacological help in conjunction with lifestyle modifications.

The intertwining of stress and heart disease is undeniable, but it is not an invincible connection. Through strategic lifestyle changes, mindful practices, support systems, and medical guidance, one can not only manage stress but also potentially prevent or mitigate its deleterious effects on the heart. As we explore further avenues for heart health, remember that nurturing your mental and emotional well-being is just as important as caring for your physical self.

Mindfulness and Stress Reduction Techniques

Navigating the complexities of heart health requires more than just understanding physical symptoms or adhering to a dietary plan. It involves a comprehensive approach to well-being that includes managing stress, which is a significant risk factor for heart disease. In this section, devoted exclusively to mindfulness and stress reduction techniques, we delve into strategies that serve as essential tools for heart health. Each of these techniques is designed to enhance your overall health and can be integrated into your lifestyle to help alleviate stress, which in turn can lower your risk of heart-related issues.

So what is mindfulness? At its core, mindfulness is a practice of being fully present in the moment, aware of where we are and what we're doing, without becoming overly reactive or overwhelmed by what's going on around us. It's about observing our thoughts and feelings from a distance, without judging them as good or bad. When applied to stress reduction, mindfulness involves techniques that quiet the mind and release tension in the body, helping you combat the negative effects stress has on your cardiovascular system.

One foundational mindfulness technique is meditation. Meditation provides a space to step away from the chaotic stimuli of everyday life and enter a state of tranquility and reflection. For heart health, just a few minutes a day devoted to meditation can decrease blood pressure, enhance sleep, and improve emotional balance. To practice, find a quiet space, close your eyes, and focus on your breath. When your mind wanders, as it will, gently bring your attention back to the rhythm of your breathing.

Another method to foster mindfulness is through focused breathing exercises. These exercises, such as deep diaphragmatic breathing, encourage full oxygen exchange and can lower the heartbeat and blood pressure, promoting calmness. Try inhaling slowly through your nose, allowing your abdomen to rise before your chest, and then exhaling thoroughly through your mouth.

Yoga, which combines physical postures, breath control, and meditation, is yet another potent stress-reducer to consider. Not only can it improve flexibility, balance, and strength, but it also offers cardiovascular benefits by relieving stress and promoting relaxation. Whether you're new or experienced, incorporating yoga into your routine a few times a week can have profound effects on your heart health.

Progressive muscle relaxation is a technique that helps relieve the tension that stress causes in the body. By systematically tensing and then relaxing different muscle groups, you become more aware of physical sensations and learn how to consciously release stress. This awareness can lower stress hormone levels, reducing strain on your heart.

Tai Chi, an ancient Chinese martial art often described as "meditation in motion," is a low-impact, slow-motion exercise where you go without pause through a series of movements. It's known for its ability to alleviate stress and anxiety, which is vital for maintaining a heart-healthy lifestyle.

Guided imagery is another form of mindful stress reduction where you visualize a peaceful setting or scenario, engaging all of your senses to immerse yourself in the experience. This technique has been linked to improved mood and reduced stress, which can have a direct effect on heart health.

The practice of gratitude can also transform your stress levels. By focusing on the positive elements in our lives, we can shift our attention away from stresses and anxieties. Maintaining a gratitude journal or simply taking time each day to acknowledge the things you're thankful for can reinforce positive emotions and contribute to a healthier heart.

Furthermore, cultivating strong social connections can lead to better stress management. Socializing can act as a buffer against stress, as it often involves shared experiences that can bring laughter, support, and joy. Building relationships with friends, family, or support groups can provide emotional comfort, which helps alleviate stress.

Adopting a mindfulness-based stress reduction (MBSR) program, which typically includes practices such as meditation, body awareness, and yoga, could be particularly effective for those dealing with heart disease. Created to reduce stress, MBSR programs are often taught in group settings and can help participants learn coping skills that improve their quality of life.

Incorporating mindfulness into your daily routine doesn't need to be daunting. You can start small—by dedicating just five minutes a day to any of these practices and gradually increasing as you become more comfortable. Unlike strenuous physical activity, mindfulness techniques are low-risk, making them an excellent option for individuals at various stages of heart disease.

It's also important to remember that while mindfulness is a powerful tool, it's not a cure-all. It works best as a component of an integrated approach to heart health, one that includes proper nutrition, regular physical activity, and medical care. By reducing stress through mindfulness, we lighten the load on our hearts, enhancing both our emotional well-being and our physiological health.

As we grasp mindfulness and integrate it into our lives, we're not just managing stress; we're breeding a profound level of consciousness that knows no bounds. This consciousness allows us to live more fully, making choices that align with our best interests, including those that support our heart health.

To conclude, stress is an inescapable part of life, but it doesn't have to dictate our health outcomes. Mindfulness and stress reduction techniques offer reprieve and recalibration for our bodies and minds, allowing us to navigate life with resilience and grace. By empowering ourselves with these tools, we sustain not just our hearts, but our holistic existence.

Chapter 9:
Navigating Healthcare
and Heart Tests

Having explored the fundamentals of heart disease, its unique manifestations in women, and the potent lifestyle changes you can adopt to bolster heart health, Chapter 9 steers you through the often-daunting terrain of the healthcare system and the vital heart tests that can illuminate your path. Empowering yourself begins with choosing healthcare providers who are not only experts in their field but also partners in your heart health journey. You'll learn how to cultivate a team that communicates clearly and involves you in decision-making processes. This chapter also delves into the assortment of essential heart health screenings and tests, from blood pressure and cholesterol levels to cutting-edge imaging techniques. All of these tools are instrumental to your quest for a resilient heart. They unlock your ability to track progress, detect potential issues before they escalate, and make informed choices that align with your health goals. As you turn the page, you're not just reading about tests and treatments; you're stepping closer to a future where you navigate healthcare with confidence and a heart that's supported by the very best that medicine has to offer.

Choosing the Right Healthcare Providers

Embarking on a journey towards better heart health warrants assembling a team of healthcare providers who not only possess the right expertise but also align with your health goals and values. The intricacy of heart disease, especially in the context of its variability between genders, necessitates a selection process as crucial as the treatment itself.

Identifying a cardiologist who specializes in women's heart health can be transformative. Research indicates that female cardiologists may offer a nuanced perspective on heart disease in women, and a more holistic approach to treatment. Ensure that your cardiologist is board-certified, which signals that they have undergone rigorous training and are up-to-date on the latest advancements in heart care.

Moreover, consider a multidisciplinary team approach. Your heart health care team might include a primary care physician, a cardiologist, a dietitian, and perhaps a fitness expert. Each plays a pivotal role; your primary care physician acts as the gatekeeper, your cardiologist as the strategist, your dietitian as the nutrition architect, and your fitness expert as the movement coach.

It's important to carefully vet any potential healthcare provider. Check their credentials and patient reviews. Additionally, take into consideration their communication style. Can they explain complex information in an understandable way? Are they an active listener, responding thoughtfully to your questions and concerns? These qualities are essential for a successful patient-provider relationship.

Accessibility is another factor to ponder. Your providers should be reasonably reachable for appointments and in cases of emergency. Telemedicine has expanded the options here, potentially making regular check-ins more convenient without sacrificing quality of care.

When discussing your treatment options, transparency around the benefits, risks, and alternatives of proposed interventions is critical. Your healthcare provider should be willing to explore all viable options, helping you make informed decisions that resonate with your lifestyle and preferences.

Additionally, take note of the support staff at healthcare practices. Nurses, physician assistants, and administrative staff's demeanor and responsiveness contribute to the overall care experience and can greatly impact the efficiency of your healthcare journey.

Consider also the importance of culturally competent care. Providers who respect and understand your cultural background, beliefs, and values can dramatically improve communication and trust, and thereby, the effectiveness of your treatment plan.

For those living with conditions beyond heart disease, finding healthcare providers who understand how comorbidities intersect is vital. A team that is capable of an integrated approach to managing multiple health concerns may better tailor your care plans.

Coordination of care among your healthcare providers is not just a convenience; it is a necessity for comprehensive care. Ensure that there are systems in place for your healthcare providers to collaborate and share information, which helps in devising a cohesive and streamlined care strategy.

Don't forget that choosing the right healthcare provider is an evolving process. As your health needs change, it may be necessary to reevaluate your team. It's crucial to remain proactive and involved in the decision-making process throughout your heart health journey.

In the end, personal comfort with your healthcare providers can make a substantial difference. Trust your instincts. If you're feeling uncertain or uncomfortable with a provider, it may be worth considering a change. Your health and well-being are paramount, and your healthcare team should be a sanctuary of support and expertise.

And finally, remember that you are the most important member of your healthcare team. Your engagement, questions, and feedback are invaluable. Choose providers who value patient empowerment and view your health journey as a partnership.

In the path to improved heart health, having the right healthcare providers is akin to having the right fuel for a vehicle; it can propel you forward, ensure smooth navigation, and ultimately, help you reach your destination of a healthier heart and a fuller life.

Essential Heart Health Screenings and Tests

Embracing a proactive approach in heart health involves understanding the screenings and tests fundamental to detecting and monitoring cardiovascular conditions—your defense arsenal in early detection, prevention, and management. An informed grasp of these screenings bolsters your ability to engage constructively with healthcare providers, ensuring thorough care calibrated to your body's needs.

Firstly, blood pressure measurement serves as a cornerstone for heart health screening. It's critical to ascertain whether your blood pressure lies within a healthy range, as elevated levels often portend risks for heart disease and stroke. Clinicians typically recommend regular monitoring—even if your blood pressure is normal—to detect any changes that might demand medical attention.

Cholesterol levels in your blood are another vital indicator. A simple blood test, often referred to as a lipid panel, will quantify total cholesterol, LDL ("bad" cholesterol), HDL ("good" cholesterol), and triglycerides. Imbalances in these numbers herald an increased risk for atherosclerosis, a primary contributor to heart attacks and strokes. Diet, lifestyle, and sometimes medication are deployed to manage undesired levels.

It's also important to screen for diabetes, as high blood sugar levels can damage blood vessels and nerves that help control the heart. The fasting plasma glucose test, the A1C test, or the oral glucose tolerance test are commonly used to check for diabetes or pre-diabetes, conditions that directly influence heart health.

Beyond these baseline tests, more sophisticated screenings may be advised based on risk factors and symptoms. An electrocardiogram (EKG or ECG) records the heart's electrical activity and can uncover various heart abnormalities, including arrhythmias and previous heart attacks that went unnoticed.

When further detail is required, an echocardiogram utilizes ultrasound waves to create images of the heart's chambers, valves, walls, and the blood vessels attached to the heart. It allows for a non-invasive peek into the pump's function and architecture, revealing problems such as heart muscle weakness or issues with the heart's structure.

Exercise stress tests gauge the heart's performance under physical exertion. Monitoring your heart's electrical activity while you walk on a treadmill or pedal a stationary bike, health care professionals understand how your heart responds under strain—an essential consideration in managing or deterring heart disease.

For those suspected of having coronary artery disease, or for those with symptoms that regular stress tests can't clarify, a nuclear stress test or a stress echocardiogram can be ordered. These tests incorporate radioactive substances or ultrasound, respectively, to provide additional insights, especially regarding blood flow to the heart.

Another advanced tool is the cardiac CT for calcium scoring, which detects calcium deposits in the coronary arteries. This non-invasive method offers clues on the susceptibility to heart attacks as it indicates plaque buildup that may narrow the arteries—a condition known as atherosclerosis.

In some scenarios, a cardiac catheterization may be performed. This procedure involves threading a thin tube through a blood vessel to the heart to check for blockages, collect biopsies, or even to help widen narrowed arteries. It serves both as a diagnostic tool and a potential interventional method.

Heart health checks aren't complete without considering inflammation markers, such as C-reactive protein (CRP), which can indicate increased risk for coronary diseases. High levels of CRP have been linked to a heightened probability of heart attack and stroke. Knowledge of one's CRP level can initiate preemptive strategies to quell inflammation.

For particular heart rhythm abnormalities like atrial fibrillation, a portable monitor like Holter monitor or a cardiac event recorder may be advised. These devices are worn for a time, continuously recording the heart's rhythm, capturing intermittent or elusive episodes that intermittent testing might miss.

An ankle-brachial index compares blood pressure in the ankle with blood pressure in the arm, which can reveal peripheral artery disease— a narrowing of blood vessels in areas other than the heart, such as legs. PAD often indicates more widespread atherosclerosis, which may affect the heart as well.

If sleep apnea is suspected as a contributing factor for heart conditions, a sleep study may be recommended. Unmanaged sleep apnea is increasingly recognized as a risk factor for high blood pressure, arrhythmias, stroke, and heart failure.

Last but not least in the array of heart health screenings is patient education. Understanding the significance, process, and implications of heart health tests empowers you to take ownership of your health. It is essential for individuals to engage actively with healthcare practitioners, inquire about screening intervals, and understand the interpretation of results. This dialogue fosters a collaborative, informed approach to the prevention and management of heart disease.

Mindful consideration of these screenings and tests underscores a broader commitment to heart health. When combined with lifestyle and dietary modifications, these vital assessments provide a comprehensive picture of your heart's condition, allowing for timely, targeted interventions. They reflect an investment in one's well-being, with profound dividends paid in longevity and quality of life.

Chapter 10:
Living with Heart Disease

Embracing life with heart disease involves adapting to a new normal—one that accommodates the necessary changes and challenges but also leaves ample room for joy, fulfilment, and personal growth. In this essential chapter, we address the holistic cycle of rehabilitation and recovery, empowering you to navigate the nuances of medications and medical interventions with informed confidence. Moreover, we delve into the fabric of emotional and social support networks, revealing how essential they are in bolstering your heart's health as much as your spirit's resilience. Let's journey together through the landscape of living with heart disease, where each step is an opportunity to enhance your wellbeing. It's about more than mere survival; it's about thriving—amidst diagnoses and treatments—garnering strength from a community of support, and learning to reshape life's priorities in a way that honors your heart's needs and your life's passions.

Rehabilitation and Recovery

As we step into the realm of rehabilitation and recovery following a heart disease diagnosis, we embrace a journey that interweaves the physical reconditioning of the heart with the nurturing of mental resilience. Rehabilitation is your path to reclaiming strength, embracing vitality, and achieving the best quality of life post-diagnosis. It is a multifaceted process that involves coordinated medical care, lifestyle adjustments, and unwavering determination.

For many, the road to recovery begins with a structured cardiac rehabilitation program. These programs cater to the unique needs of each individual, incorporating exercise training, education on heart-healthy living, and counseling to reduce stress and improve emotional health. The goal is to establish a foundation for long-term heart health and to equip you with the tools to manage your condition effectively.

Exercise is a cornerstone of cardiac rehabilitation, designed to fortify the heart and improve stamina. The notion of pushing one's body following a cardiac event may seem daunting; however, a gradual and supervised regimen can enhance circulation, reduce the risk of future heart complications, and uplift spirits. The key is to engage in moderate-intensity activities that you enjoy, which can lead to a more active and fulfilling life.

Educating yourself about heart disease is another integral component of recovery. Knowledge empowers you to make informed decisions about your treatment and lifestyle. Understanding how to navigate dietary choices, recognize warning signs of complications, and adhere to prescribed medication regimens can transform the quality of your life post-heart disease.

Nutrition plays a pivotal role in cardiac rehabilitation. Adopting a heart-smart diet rich in whole foods, lean proteins, and abundant in fruits and vegetables can assist in controlling weight, cholesterol, and blood pressure. Your diet should become your ally in the battle against heart disease, fueling your body with the nutrients necessary for repair and vitality.

Stress management is equally important for a holistic recovery. Chronic stress can have a perplexing effect on heart health, making stress reduction techniques such as mindfulness, deep breathing exercises, or yoga invaluable elements of your rehabilitation program. Such practices can enhance emotional well-being and further fortify your heart against stress-induced damage.

Monitoring your progress with regular check-ups and open dialogue with your healthcare team is critical. These professionals can help track your recovery trajectory, adjusting treatments as needed and providing reassurance along the way. Remember, the relationship with your healthcare providers should be a collaborative one, where you are the central contributor to your healing journey.

Medications may be a necessary component of your recovery, aiming to prevent recurrence of heart events, control symptoms, and improve your heart's functioning. Understanding and adhering to your medication regime is non-negotiable. They are the silent guardians of your heart, working behind the scenes to maintain your health.

Emotional support plays an unsung but vital role in recovery. From structured support groups to the embrace of family and friends, surrounding yourself with a positive support network can have a transformative impact on your rehabilitation journey. Emotional and social support not only provides comfort but also promotes adherence to healthy behaviors.

Sleep, often overlooked, is a powerful rehabilitative ally. Achieving restorative sleep can boost heart health, enhance mood and cognitive function, and promote overall well-being. Treat your sleep environment and routines as sacred, prioritizing them as much as diet and exercise.

Quitting smoking, if applicable, is another critical step in cardiac recovery. Smoking cessation is a challenge, yet it is one of the most impactful ways to reduce the risk of further heart damage. With the right tools and support, the journey to being smoke-free is within your grasp.

Setting realistic goals is a strategy to keep you motivated and on track. Recovery is personal, and what works for one person may not suit another. Celebrate the small victories, like taking a flight of stairs without shortness of breath or cooking a heart-healthy meal from scratch. These milestones are the building blocks of a resilient heart.

Understanding that recovery can be cyclical rather than linear allows you to manage expectations and develop resilience. There may be setbacks, but each one teaches a lesson, further arming you with the experience to navigate your heart health with grace and wisdom.

Lastly, consider this journey as an investment in your future. The habits you form, the knowledge you gain, and the support you nurture all contribute to a stronger, more vibrant heart. It's a new beginning, an opportunity to live with heart health as a priority, gifting you not just years to your life, but life to your years.

In closing, rehabilitation and recovery are not merely about surviving heart disease; they're about thriving despite it. This chapter doesn't mark the end but the continuation of a commitment to a heart-smart lifestyle that is both enriching and life-affirming. Embrace each step of this rehabilitation with courage and optimism, for your heart is resilient, and so are you.

Medications and Medical Interventions

When facing heart disease, understanding the role of medications and medical interventions is essential. These can serve as life-saving measures and ways to improve quality of life. Here we unfold the vital importance of medical therapies and procedures which work in conjunction with lifestyle changes to manage heart conditions effectively.

Medical therapy begins with a solid foundation of medications designed to treat various aspects of heart disease. Statins, for example, are instrumental in managing cholesterol levels. They function by inhibiting an enzyme involved in cholesterol production, thereby reducing the risk of atherosclerosis – a primary cause of heart attacks and strokes.

Moreover, blood pressure medications such as ACE inhibitors or beta-blockers are commonly prescribed for hypertension, an insidious condition that can lead to heart failure and kidney disease if not controlled. These drugs can lessen the workload on the heart and expand blood vessels, making it easier for the heart to pump blood.

For those with abnormal heart rhythms, antiarrhythmics and anticoagulants play a critical role. The irregular heartbeats of conditions like atrial fibrillation can cause blood clots, which may lead to stroke. Anticoagulants help prevent clot formation, while antiarrhythmics work to restore a normal heart rhythm.

Individuals dealing with heart failure often turn to diuretics and ACE inhibitors. Diuretics help reduce fluid buildup in the body, alleviating symptoms such as edema and shortness of breath. ACE inhibitors can improve survival after a heart attack by preventing further weakening of the heart muscles.

In cases of severe heart disease, surgical interventions may be necessary. Coronary artery bypass grafting (CABG), where arteries or veins from other parts of the body are used to bypass clogged arteries, improves blood flow to the heart. This surgery, while significant, can greatly enhance a patient's life expectancy and quality of life.

Another common intervention is the placement of stents during angioplasty. A stent is a small tube that is inserted into a narrowed artery to keep it open and allow blood to flow more freely, thus reducing the chance of a heart attack.

Pacemakers and defibrillators are devices implanted to control or correct abnormal heart rhythms. While a pacemaker can ensure the heart beats at a regular pace, an implantable cardioverter defibrillator (ICD) can detect and stop life-threatening arrhythmias by delivering a shock to the heart.

Innovations in medical technology have led to transcatheter aortic valve replacement (TAVR) for patients with aortic valve stenosis who are not suitable candidates for traditional open-heart surgery. Through a small incision, a replacement valve is guided to the heart, offering a minimally invasive option with quicker recovery times.

Heart disease treatment may also involve the use of clot-busting drugs, known as thrombolytics, which are used in emergency situations to dissolve blood clots that are blocking the coronary arteries during a heart attack, restoring blood flow to the heart muscle.

Even though these medications and interventions can be lifesaving, they are most effective when paired with lifestyle strategies such as a heart-healthy diet, regular exercise, stress management, and quitting smoking. It's a collaborative effort between patient and healthcare provider to create a comprehensive plan tailored to the individual's needs.

Medication adherence is a crucial aspect of heart disease management. Noncompliance can lead to worsening of the condition and increase the risk of hospitalization. Patients must understand their medications' purposes, the importance of taking them as prescribed, and potential side effects to watch for.

Patients should also be aware of novel medical therapies that emerge as research progresses. Breakthroughs in biotechnologies such as gene and stem cell therapies are on the horizon, potentially offering new ways to repair damaged heart tissue and restore heart function.

Medical interventions and medications are not without risks and potential side effects, which is why patient education and regular follow-ups with healthcare providers are paramount to monitor progress and make necessary adjustments. Remember, the combined powers of medical science and personal commitment to health can work wonders on the heart.

In conclusion, the array of medications and medical interventions available today means that heart disease is no longer an automatic death sentence. With knowledge, support, and the right mix of treatments, many with heart disease continue to lead fulfilling lives. Let these advancements empower you to take proactive steps in your heart health journey, aligning medical intervention with lifestyle choices for optimal wellbeing.

Emotional and Social Support Networks

In facing heart disease or recovery after a cardiovascular event, the role of emotional support from family, friends, and peers cannot be over-emphasized. Humans are inherently social beings and the comfort derived from feeling understood and cared for can greatly improve one's outlook and motivation for health.

Living with heart disease can be a profound challenge, one that requires not only medical intervention but emotional sustenance. Such support isn't merely comforting; it's known to have tangible benefits for heart health. Establishing and maintaining robust emotional and social support networks is a vital component in managing your heart health. These networks serve as an essential lifeline, providing both practical assistance and psychological fortitude.

Support networks may comprise family members who accompany you to appointments, friends who offer a listening ear, or community groups focused on heart health. Each interaction within these networks can help dispel the clouds of isolation that often accompany chronic illness, and instead foster a sense of connection and shared experience.

You might find solace in starting conversations with loved ones about your health journey. It's important to communicate your needs clearly and to set boundaries where necessary. Sharing your experiences, fears, and successes with those close to you can create deeper bonds and a mutual understanding, further aiding your recovery and management of heart disease.

It's not uncommon to feel a sense of pride and independence, which might discourage you from reaching out for help. However, allowing others to provide support is not an admission of weakness, but rather a strategy for strengthening your mental and emotional resilience. Social support can act as a buffer against the stress that so negatively impacts heart health, and it can also provide a source of positive reinforcement as you make lifestyle changes.

Research has consistently shown that individuals with stronger social support tend to have better health outcomes. When dealing with the pressures of heart disease, having someone to talk to can lessen anxiety and depression. These emotional states are not only distressing, but they can also exacerbate heart problems and hinder recovery. Engaging with others provides distraction, levity, and the reassurance that you're not alone in your struggles.

Furthermore, becoming part of support groups, specifically tailored for those with heart disease, can be immensely beneficial. There, you can exchange stories, advice, and encouragement with others who truly understand what you are going through. The solidarity found in support groups often fosters feelings of empowerment and hope.

These gatherings can be found through local hospitals, wellness centers, or online communities. Some are led by healthcare professionals, while others are peer-led. The format doesn't matter as much as the fact that you are taking part in a collective endeavor to improve heart health through shared experiences.

Embracing social interactions and maintaining relationships can be particularly vital as one ages or when living with a chronic condition like heart disease. Participating in community events, volunteering, or even casual social engagements can keep your spirits high and your mind engaged. Socially active individuals are often more likely to stay physically active too, which is a key factor in managing heart disease.

If face-to-face interactions are limited, technology offers new avenues for connection. Utilize video calls, social media, or specialized apps designed to connect people with similar health challenges. The availability of such technology ensures that even those who are homebound or living in remote areas can benefit from the power of social support.

Partnerships with healthcare providers are also a form of support. By building a trusting relationship with your healthcare team, you create another layer of emotional and social support. This partnership is integral to managing heart disease effectively, as your providers can offer not only medical expertise but also encouragement and understanding.

When tapping into social networks, it's important to recognize and accept the diverse ways in which people express care and concern. While some may be great listeners, others may excel in providing practical help like cooking meals or assisting with household chores. Acknowledging the value of these varied forms of support is key to fostering a comprehensive support system.

The journey with heart disease is not one you have to walk alone. Seek out connections, communicate openly, and allow yourself the comfort of knowing that your emotional and social networks are cornerstones of your heart health strategy. They are lifelines that can make navigating the challenges of heart disease not only more bearable but also more successful.

Lastly, remember to offer your own support to others when you can. What you contribute to your support networks not only helps others but also enhances your sense of purpose and connection. In the interconnectedness of our experiences, there is strength - strength that is vital to both the heart and the soul.

Chapter 11:
Prevention and Early
Detection Strategies

Moving seamlessly from understanding the impact of living with heart disease, we now transition to the proactive realm of prevention and early detection strategies. It's imperative that we embrace lifestyle choices that not only thwart the progression of heart disease but also fortify our defenses against its onset. Marrying the principles of vigilant self-care—like a balanced diet replete with heart-boosting nutrients and regular physical activity—with the precision of medical screenings can create a formidable shield against cardiovascular afflictions. Knowing when and how often to undergo heart health assessments is a cornerstone of this strategy. By cultivating a vigilant partnership with healthcare providers, we ensure that any whisper of abnormality in our heart's rhythm or cadence is caught before it crescendos into a clamor—a feat that significantly elevates our odds of sustaining a vigorous, thriving life.

Lifestyle Choices for Prevention

Leading a heart-healthy lifestyle is a potent defense against heart disease. What you do in your daily life has a significant impact on your heart health, and making conscientious lifestyle choices can serve as your armor in the fight against cardiovascular disease. This section explores how taking charge of your lifestyle can dramatically reduce your risk of heart complications.

Firstly, consider tobacco usage. If you smoke or use tobacco products, it's time to quit. The chemicals in tobacco can damage your heart and blood vessels, leading to narrowing of the arteries (atherosclerosis), which can ultimately cause a heart attack. No amount of smoking is safe, and quitting is paramount. Even exposure to secondhand smoke can be damaging, so it's crucial to avoid it whenever possible.

Maintaining a healthy weight plays a critical role in preventing heart disease. Excess weight can lead to conditions that increase your chances of heart disease — including high blood pressure, high cholesterol, and type 2 diabetes. Even a small weight loss can be beneficial. Reducing your weight by just 3% to 5% can help decrease certain fats in your blood (triglycerides), lower your blood sugar, and reduce your risk of type 2 diabetes.

Eating a diet rich in vegetables, fruits, whole grains, and lean proteins can help protect your heart. Limiting certain fats you eat is also important. Reducing the amount of saturated and trans fats can reduce your blood cholesterol and lower your risk of coronary artery disease. A high blood cholesterol level can lead to a buildup of plaques in your arteries, which can increase the risk of heart attack and stroke.

Physical activity is a cornerstone of heart health. Aim for at least 150 minutes of moderate aerobic activity or 75 minutes of vigorous aerobic activity each week, or a combination of moderate and vigorous activity. Also, incorporate muscle-strengthening activities two days a week. Physical activity can help you control your weight and reduce your chances of developing other conditions that may put a strain on your heart.

Limiting alcohol intake can also be beneficial. Drinking too much alcohol can raise your blood pressure. It also adds extra calories, which may cause weight gain — both of which are risks factors for heart disease. Men should have no more than two alcoholic drinks per day, and women no more than one.

Getting enough quality sleep is essential for good heart health. Sleep deprivation can put you at an increased risk for cardiovascular disease, regardless of your age or other health habits. Strive for 7 to 9 hours of quality sleep per night, and consult a healthcare provider if you have chronic sleep problems.

Managing stress in healthful ways can mitigate its negative impact on the heart. Chronic stress can contribute to heart disease, especially if it leads to smoking, overeating, or other unhealthy behaviors. Finding healthy ways to manage stress—such as physical activity, relaxation exercises, or meditation—can help improve your health.

Regular health screenings for blood pressure, blood sugar, cholesterol, and more can detect heart-related issues early on. These tests can identify risk factors that can be managed through lifestyle changes or medication, thus reducing the heart disease risk.

Don't underestimate the power of daily habits over your heart health. Simple actions such as taking the stairs instead of the elevator, parking further away from store entrances, or incorporating short walks into your breaks can contribute to your cardiovascular fitness.

Additionally, oral health may be a window to your overall health. Some research suggests that the bacteria that cause gum disease can also increase your risk of heart disease. So, brush and floss your teeth daily and get regular dental checkups.

Environmental factors like air pollution can affect your heart health. It's important to check the Air Quality Index (AQI) in your area and limit outdoor activities when pollution levels are high to reduce your exposure to harmful particles that can affect your heart health.

Limit your intake of sodium, which can contribute to high blood pressure, a risk factor for cardiovascular disease. The American Heart Association recommends no more than 2,300 milligrams (mg) a day and moving toward an ideal limit of no more than 1,500 mg per day for most adults.

Stay informed and proactive about your health. Understanding your own medical history and risk factors is crucial. Discuss your family history with your healthcare provider and consider genetic testing if recommended to understand your predisposition towards heart disease. Knowledge is power, and staying informed is a proactive way to manage your heart health.

Lastly, build a support network. Whether it's family, friends, or a support group for those with heart disease, having people to share the journey can make a significant difference in your success. Emotional support can help you maintain the motivation you need to care for your heart.

Adopting these heart-healthy lifestyle choices doesn't have to be overwhelming. Rather than making large changes all at once, start with small steps that you can build on over time. Remember, every positive choice you make can contribute to your overall heart health and quality of life. Embrace these choices with confidence and commitment, knowing that you are taking control of your heart health and setting the stage for a healthier future.

The Role of Regular Screenings

Embarking on the path to a healthier heart is a commitment that requires not just lifestyle changes, but also a proactive approach to monitoring one's health. Regular screenings play a pivotal role in this journey, serving as both compass and map to guide individuals through the terrain of heart health maintenance and disease prevention.

At the heart—pun intended—of regular screenings is early detection. Catching heart disease in its earliest stages exponentially increases the chances for successful intervention and treatment. These screenings, when harmonized with a person's family history, age, and overall health, can unveil hidden risks and provide an early warning system that is critical for initiating life-saving measures.

Moreover, consider the dynamic nature of the cardiovascular system and the fact that risk factors can evolve over time. Regular check-ups ensure that both static and dynamic risk factors are accounted for, offering an updated assessment of heart health. Conditions like hypertension and high cholesterol, notorious for their covert existence, can be detected and managed before they escalate into more severe complications.

Screenings often begin with blood pressure measurements, a simple yet potent diagnostic tool. Hypertension is the harbinger of potential heart-related woes and warrants vigilant monitoring. Determining one's baseline blood pressure and watching for upward trends over time can trigger interventions that specifically target reductions in blood pressure.

Cholesterol profiling is another mainstay of heart health screenings. Lipid panels render a detailed account of the types of fats coursing through one's bloodstream, distinguishing between the benevolent and the troublesome. Recognizing unhealthy patterns in cholesterol levels can incite dietary and lifestyle modifications, and when necessary, medical management.

Diabetes, with its deleterious effects on blood vessels, requires careful monitoring to keep its associated risks at bay. Blood glucose screenings serve as a gauge for detecting prediabetes or diabetes, both of which constitute significant risk factors for heart disease. Controlling blood sugar levels is imperative for heart health and is best accomplished through a synergy of screenings, diet, exercise, and potential medication.

Additional screening tests may include electrocardiograms to elucidate the heart's electrical activity, or more sophisticated imaging like echocardiograms, which provide intricate details about the heart's structure and function. These tests delve deeper into the heart's condition, revealing silent threats that may have been brewing without symptoms.

Treadmill stress tests, too, play their part by measuring the heart's response to exertion. Uneven heart rhythms or inadequate blood flow detected during these tests can indicate the presence of coronary artery disease or other conditions that may otherwise go unnoticed.

For certain high-risk individuals, including those with a family history of heart disease, advanced screenings like coronary calcium scans may be recommended. These scans seek out calcified deposits in the arteries—an early sign of coronary artery disease—and quantify their burden, thus giving a tangible metric to measure and monitor over time.

When considering the comprehensive approach to heart health, it's essential to recognize that regular screenings are both advantageous and cost-effective. By identifying problems early, individuals can avoid the higher costs and increased morbidity associated with advanced heart disease. In this sense, investing in regular screenings is not only a health decision but a sound financial strategy as well.

Participating in regular screenings also creates an invaluable partnership between the individual and healthcare professionals. It facilitates open dialogue, shared decision-making, and the development of a tailored health plan that evolves with the patient's changing needs. Such collaboration is integral for adapting to the nuances of each unique heart health journey.

While screenings are indeed critical, it's imperative to remember that they are not a standalone solution. They should complement a heart-focused lifestyle that includes balanced nutrition, regular exercise, stress management, and the avoidance of harmful substances such as tobacco.

What then is our course of action? First, we must schedule and adhere to recommended screening intervals. Second, engage with the results of these screenings—understand them, act upon them, and make them catalysts for sustained heart health activities.

Ultimately, the narrative of our health is authored through everyday actions and decisions. Screenings are one of the many chapters that illustrate our commitment to actively preserving the vitality and functionality of our hearts. Embrace these preventive measures with the understanding that they lead to more than mere longevity; they point toward a quality of life that is rich in fulfillment and brimming with potential.

As we transition to our next section, let us carry forward the knowledge of how regular screenings reveal much about our health's current story, while also dictating the arc of its future chapters. Screenings are our strategic ally in the quest for a robust and resilient heart, and our diligence in scheduling and responding to them will chart the course for heart health outcomes that favor vitality, wellness, and life.

Chapter 12:
Empowering Stories of
Strength and Survival

In the heart of every struggle lies a story of resilience and in Chapter 12, we share those narratives that echo the triumph of the human spirit over the hardships of heart disease. Engage with the lived experiences of individuals who've faced the foreboding diagnosis and emerged stronger, fusing their newfound wisdom with a zest for life that's both contagious and affirming. Their powerful testimonials serve as beacons of hope, illuminating the path for those navigating their own recovery journeys. Each anecdote underscores the boundless potential within us to overcome adversity through courage, informed decision-making, and unwavering support networks. Take heart in these lessons of perseverance, allowing them to guide you towards a life marked not just by survival, but by thriving health and happiness.

Inspirational Testimonials

Within the heartbeats of survivors and thrivers, lies the pulsating rhythm of hope and transformation. The journey through the landscape of heart disease is unique for each person, yet there's a common thread in the tapestry of their experiences—an unwavering spirit and a determination to thrive despite the odds. The individuals who have graciously shared their stories here provide not just inspiration but tangible evidence that change is possible, and a healthier heart can often be reclaimed through commitment, support, and deliberate life-style adjustments.

Take Leah, for instance, who at the age of 52, found herself in the clutches of a heart attack. It was a wake-up call that she couldn't ignore. Leah's journey to recovery was paved with the stones of dietary change, regular exercise, and a new outlook on stress management. Her story isn't just about survival; it's about flourishing—finding delight in morning walks and joy in the colorful abundance of her vegetable garden.

Or consider Michael, a seasoned firefighter, who learned that even heroes are vulnerable. After facing a frightening diagnosis of hyper-trophic cardiomyopathy, Michael decided to use his fighting spirit to battle for his health. He revamped his diet, prioritized sleep, and em-braced yoga, an activity he once thought was not for him. It's his belief in continual self-improvement and adaptation that fuels his progress.

Then there's Jasmine, who inherited more than her mother's smile; she inherited the risk for heart disease. Yet, knowledge was power for Jasmine. She educated herself, advocated for her health, and took pre-ventive measures seriously. Seeing her children grow up with the understanding of a heart-healthy lifestyle is her greatest reward and tes-tament to her perseverance.

Jorge's story is equally compelling. He battled high blood pressure and cholesterol, flirting with danger, until his daughter's earnest plea shifted his perspective. Jorge's transformation involved learning to cook meals that nurtured his heart and forming bonds over brisk fami-ly walks. His new lifestyle choices became cherished family activities, reinforcing the power of support and love in recovery.

Emma, a young professional, tackled her heart disease with the precision of a CEO. She set goals, created action plans, and surrounded herself with a team of healthcare professionals who understood her holistic approach to health. Emma's tale serves as an impressive blue-print for others about the critical importance of comprehensive healthcare navigation.

Raj found courage in the adversity of a stroke. Though the road to rehabilitation was daunting, he discovered resilience he never knew he had. With the encouragement of therapists and the unwavering company of his pet dog, Raj learned to celebrate each victory, no matter how small, redefining his limits with every step forward.

Carol, who always put herself last, faced heart disease after decades of neglecting her well-being. Her journey underlines the necessity of self-care—a lesson she now shares with every woman she meets. By placing her health on her priority list, Carol found a new chapter of life, vibrant and fuller than she ever imagined.

Dan's story sheds light on the transformative effects of mindfulness on heart health. After surviving a coronary artery blockage, Dan embraced meditation to manage his stress levels. It wasn't long before this practice spilled into other areas of his life, leading to more thoughtful eating habits and a profound sense of inner calm.

Sophia's brush with death came unexpectedly during a run—a hobby she believed was her safeguard against illness. Her collapse from undiagnosed arrhythmia became the catalyst for advocating for routine screenings—especially for those who seem the picture of health. Sophia is now a champion for heart health awareness in her community.

Bill, a retired school teacher, faced the enormity of congestive heart failure. His determination saw him through multiple hospital visits and the complexity of treatment regimens. Despite the challenges, Bill's spirit never wavered. Through his educational approach, he manages his condition with discipline and an insatiable appetite for learning about his health.

And there's Maya, whose congenital heart defect didn't prevent her from climbing mountains—both literal and metaphorical. Maya's vigor and passion for adventure didn't just inspire her to recover; they compelled her to help others with similar conditions, exemplifying the capacity of the human heart to not only endure but to inspire.

Derek, who quietly battled depression along with heart disease, found solace in reconnecting with his passion for music. By channeling his emotions through creativity, he not only nurtured his mental health but discovered the therapeutic power of expression on his cardiovascular well-being.

Katie, a mother of three, faced the terrifying reality of her heart's vulnerability when she experienced cardiac arrest. Her recovery was supported by technology—implantable devices—and the comfort of her children's laughter, a reminder of all the beautiful reasons to fight for health and life.

And let us not forget Tom, whose heart transplant journey shines a light on the miracles of modern medicine and the depth of human generosity. Tom's gratitude towards his donor is a daily reminder of the preciousness of each heartbeat, the gift of time, and the importance of giving and receiving compassion.

The narratives of these individuals encapsulate more than their hardships; they are shining beacons of hope, illustrating that the path to heart health is tread one step at a time. Through their stories, we're reminded of the intrinsic strength found in the shared human experience, the promise of renewal, and the exceptional fortitude of the heart.

Lessons Learned and the Road to Recovery

Each journey through heart disease is a personal narrative that weaves lessons of resilience, adaptation, and rebirth. For many, surviving a heart event can be a profound wake-up call, signaling the need for sweeping life changes. It's a road that demands courage, but it's also paved with invaluable lessons and myriad opportunities for growth.

Understanding that recovery transcends the physical is the first step on this road. Rebuilding a heart that's been through trauma isn't just about restoring its physical function—it's about healing and strengthening the whole person. Embracing a balanced diet, engaging in regular physical activity, and managing stress are not merely treatments; they're transformative practices that can renew your life.

Educating oneself about heart disease is as empowering as it's enlightening. Knowledge is instrumental in making informed decisions about one's health, fostering a sense of control and ownership over the recovery process. Furthermore, education dismantles fear, replacing it with understanding and the ability to act proactively in preserving one's well-being.

Another pivotal lesson arises from recognizing and respecting the mind-body connection. The health of the heart is intimately tied to mental and emotional states. Techniques that foster mindfulness can be powerful allies in managing stress and emotional turbulence, thus contributing to both mental and a heart-healthy recovery.

It's crucial to acknowledge the role of a solid support network. Be it family, friends, or support groups, having a network provides a buffer against the loneliness that can accompany illness. These networks don't just offer emotional comfort; they can also be sources of practical advice and motivation.

Medication and medical intervention are not standalone solutions – they're part of a larger wellness puzzle. It's essential to adopt a holistic approach to health, where treatments are complemented with lifestyle changes to optimize recovery and prevent future events.

Those on the path to recovery often learn the value of patience. Healing is not instant. It's a process that unfolds in its own time, and understanding this helps in setting realistic goals and expectations. A gradual, step-by-step approach ensures a more sustainable recovery.

Recovery also teaches the importance of adaptability. Life after a heart event may require new routines and altered priorities. It's about finding what works for you, your body, and your circumstances, and being prepared to make necessary adjustments.

Importantly, those who have traversed this path stress the significance of regular screenings and check-ups. Early detection of any deviations from the recovery plan allows for timely interventions, which can significantly improve long-term outcomes.

Appreciating life's fragility often leads to profound personal transformation. This newfound gratitude can catalyze positive life changes, inspire others, and sometimes even lead to a reevaluation of one's purpose and goals. It's an impetus to live more consciously and meaningfully.

Many who walk the road to recovery become advocates for heart health, driven by the desire to share their experiences and knowledge. Their stories can be instrumental in raising awareness and inspiring others to take action in their heart health journeys.

Listening to one's own body becomes a vital skill learned through recovery. Tuning into the subtle cues it provides allows for early recognition of potential issues and can guide daily choices in nutrition, activity, and stress management.

Throughout the recovery journey, emotional resilience takes on a new significance. Those who have faced heart disease learn the power of a positive mindset—a perspective that embraces life's challenges as opportunities for growth, rather than insurmountable obstacles.

Ultimately, this road is about rediscovering joy and building a life that feels full and vibrant, even in the face of heart disease. Recovering heart patients learn to find joy in the simplicity of a walk, the nourishment of a meal, or the comfort of connection—simple pleasures that feed the heart in more ways than one.

The lessons learned on the road to recovery are as diverse as the individuals who travel it. However, they coalesce around common themes of empowerment, resilience, and hope. As you face your own journey with heart disease, bear in mind that each step taken, no matter how small, is a triumph. With each personal story of recovery, there's a treasure trove of lessons to be unearthed, not just for living with heart disease, but for living well in every sense.

Online Review Request for This Book

If you've found inspiration and practical guidance in "Empowering Stories of Strength and Survival," please consider sharing your thoughts by leaving an online review to help others on their heart health journey.

Chapter 13:
Your Heart-Smart Future

The journey through the labyrinth of heart health information ends here, but your heart-smart future is just beginning. In the previous chapters, we've explored the complexities of heart disease, particularly in women, the subtleties of symptoms to be vigilant about, and the risk factors that play a critical role in the health of your cardiovascular system. Now, let's focus on distilling this knowledge into a pragmatic blueprint for a future where your heart health is prioritized.

The anatomy of your heart is remarkable, crafted to sustain you with every beat. By understanding how heart disease develops over time, you've armed yourself with the intelligence to thwart its progression. Recognize that the power of knowledge is the first step in transforming your wellbeing. From here on, every choice you make has the potential to be an informed one, contributing to a fortified heart.

Let's talk about strokes—the silent killers that demand our attention. Through your commitment to learning the FAST protocol and recognizing stroke signs, you've maximized your preparedness. This readiness isn't just for your benefit; it extends to your loved ones and your community at large.

Managing risk factors within your control, such as eliminating smoking, maintaining a balanced diet, and keeping a vigilant watch on blood pressure, are all actions within your reach. The essence of controllable risk factors is that they can be modified, shaped, and adapted to serve your heart's demands.

101

While certain risks are etched in the stone of your genetic code or tied to the ticking clock of age, they serve not as deterrents but as motivators. They remind us that while we can't outrun every aspect of our biology, we can make strides in mitigating risks through lifestyle alterations and a steadfast partnership with healthcare professionals.

What does a heart-smart diet look like? It's replete with nutrient-dense foods, brimming with life-giving antioxidants, and balanced with the right types of fats and sugars. It's not just about restrictions; it's about embracing a cornucopia of choices that delight the senses while nourishing the heart.

Your heart thrives on movement, and your commitment to fitness isn't a fleeting trend; it's a cornerstone of your heart's vitality. Whether it's a spirited walk, a soothing yoga routine, or energetic strength training, each drop of sweat is a testament to your heart's resilience.

Never underestimate the power of the mind-heart connection. Stress and mental health are as integral to your heart's welfare as any medication or diet. Sharpen your mindfulness and stress reduction techniques as these are the invisible armor against life's slings and arrows, safeguarding your heart from the stresses that would seek to undermine it.

You've navigated the healthcare maze and now stand equipped to make informed decisions. The appropriate screenings and tests aren't just a part of a routine; they're your sentinel guardians, offering early warnings and ensuring that your heart is shielded from foreseeable harm.

For those living with heart disease, there's a community and network stretching out their hands in solidarity. Rehabilitation, medication, and interventions are part of a collective effort to bring you back to a place of strength. Remember, the heart's ability to recover is remarkable, and your emotional and social well-being is integral to that process.

Prevention is your torch in the fog of potential health challenges. You are tasked with the duty of maintaining regular screenings and choosing daily habits that align with your heart's needs. This is your proactive strike against heart disease, and it's a strike made stronger by an unwavering commitment to your health.

As we reflect on the empowering stories of strength and survival, understand that these narratives are shared not just for inspiration but as a collective wisdom to draw upon. The road to recovery is not a solitary one; it's paved by the footsteps of those who've walked before you, guiding you toward a resilient heart.

Your heart-smart future isn't a vision; it's a tangible, achievable reality. Every adjustment to your diet, each step of exercise, and all the silent moments in meditation are the building blocks of a fortress around your heart. The key lies in consistency—small, dedicated actions repeated over time forge an unbreakable chain of habits that protect and enhance your cardiovascular health.

In this dynamic, ever-evolving landscape of heart health, your education doesn't end with the last page of this book. Appendix A, B, and C offer a treasure trove of resources, recipes, and exercise guides to keep you engaged and informed. Let these tools be your companions, as you continue to learn, grow, and adapt in your heart-smart journey.

Embrace this heart-smart future with confidence, knowing that each beat of your heart is a drumroll to a life lived with intention, care, and profound respect for the miraculous organ that keeps you moving forward. Wear your knowledge as your armor and wield your choices as your weapons in the fight for heart health. Here's to a future where your heart is not just surviving but thriving—a future that starts now.

Appendix A: Heart Health Resources

Embarking on the journey to bolster your heart health signifies a powerful commitment to your overall well-being. As you soak up the knowledge within these pages about heart disease and its complexities, it's pivotal to have practical tools and resources at your disposal. To aid in your pursuit of a heart-healthy lifestyle, Appendix A has been meticulously curated to provide a compass that guides you towards reliable information, support, and expert advice.

Online Resources and Websites

Knowledge is power, and the internet is a treasure trove of it. However, ensuring that you're getting accurate and helpful information is essential. Here's a list of credible online resources:

- The American Heart Association (heart.org) - Offers extensive information on heart disease, life-saving tips, and community initiatives.

- The Centers for Disease Control and Prevention (cdc.gov/heartdisease) - Provides statistics, facts, and educational materials on heart health.

- WomenHeart: The National Coalition for Women with Heart Disease (womenheart.org) - Focused on the unique challenges of women's heart health.

Books and Literature

In addition to this transformative reading experience, expanding your library with other insightful books can fortify your understanding and commitment:

1. "Prevent and Reverse Heart Disease" by Caldwell B. Esselstyn Jr., M.D. - An exploration into the role of diet in managing heart disease.

2. "The South Beach Heart Program" by Arthur Agatston, M.D. - A notable cardiologist offers his expertise on beating heart disease.

Support Groups and Forums

Remember, you're not treading this path alone. Engage with communities and forums where you can share your story, listen to others, and find solace in shared experiences:

- Mended Hearts (mendedhearts.org) - A community-based support network for heart patients and their families.

- Heart Disease Support Group on Inspire (inspire.com/groups/heart-disease) - Connect with others affected by heart disease, share experiences and offer support.

Apps and Technology

Leverage the power of technology to manage your heart health with these innovative apps that track everything from your diet to your exercise routines:

1. MyFitnessPal - A helpful calorie counting tool that integrates with your fitness tracking devices.

2. Blood Pressure Monitor - An app that logs and analyses your blood pressure readings over time.

Professional Organizations and Societies

Establish connections with professional organizations dedicated to fighting heart disease through research, education, and advocacy:

- The Heart Foundation (theheartfoundation.org) - Their mission is to save lives by educating the public about heart disease, promoting early detection, and fostering research.

- Heart Rhythm Society (hrsonline.org) - Focuses on the study and treatment of heart rhythm disorders.

Now, with this arsenal of resources at your fingertips, embrace the empowerment that comes from being well-informed. With each step you take, you're not only advocating for your own heart health but also serving as a beacon of inspiration for others on a similar journey. Your heart is the engine of your life; protect it with the same fervor with which you live each day. Continue to seek out knowledge, support, and new ways to thrive, and let the beat of your heart be the rhythm to your life's most beautiful song.

Appendix B:
Recipes for a Heart-Healthy Diet

Nourishing your heart is one of the most vital steps you can take on your journey towards optimal wellness. Within these pages, you'll find thoughtfully crafted recipes that cater to the nourishment and care your heart deserves. Each recipe is brimming with heart-healthy ingredients that aim to reduce inflammation, lower cholesterol levels, and support overall cardiovascular health.

Embrace the adventure of trying new flavors and ingredients, understanding that with each bite, you're making a choice that supports your wellbeing. Let's transform the way we think about food, from a mere necessity to a joyful practice of love and care for our hearts.

Sweet Potato and Black Bean Quinoa Bowl

Ingredients:

- 1 large sweet potato, peeled and diced
- 1 cup quinoa, rinsed
- 2 cups water
- 1 can black beans, drained and rinsed
- 1 avocado, sliced
- 1 cup fresh spinach, chopped
- 2 tbsp olive oil

- 1 tsp ground cumin
- Salt and pepper to taste

Instructions:

1. Preheat oven to 400°F (200°C).

2. Toss sweet potato chunks with 1 tablespoon olive oil, cumin, salt, and pepper. Spread on a baking sheet and roast for 25 minutes, or until tender.

3. In a medium saucepan, combine quinoa and water. Bring to a boil, then cover and simmer for 15 minutes, or until water is absorbed.

4. Fluff quinoa with a fork, then mix in black beans and spinach. The residual heat will wilt the spinach.

5. Divide the quinoa mixture into bowls, top with roasted sweet potato, and garnish with avocado slices.

6. Drizzle with the remaining olive oil, if desired, before serving.

Grilled Salmon with a Lemon-Dill Yogurt Sauce

Ingredients:

- 4 salmon fillets, skin-on
- 2 tbsp extra-virgin olive oil
- 1 lemon, zest and juice
- Salt and freshly ground black pepper to taste
- 1 cup Greek yogurt
- 2 tbsp fresh dill, chopped

- 1 garlic clove, minced

Instructions:

1. Preheat grill to medium-high heat.

2. Brush salmon fillets with olive oil and season with salt, pepper, and half of the lemon zest.

3. Grill salmon skin-side down for 5-6 minutes, then flip and cook for an additional 3-4 minutes or until desired doneness.

4. While the salmon cooks, combine Greek yogurt, dill, minced garlic, remaining lemon zest, and lemon juice in a small bowl. Stir to combine and season with salt and pepper to taste.

5. Once salmon is cooked, plate each fillet and drizzle with the lemon-dill yogurt sauce.

Heart-Healthy Berry and Walnut Oatmeal

Ingredients:

- 1 cup old-fashioned rolled oats
- 2 cups water or almond milk
- A pinch of salt
- 1/2 cup mixed berries (blueberries, raspberries, strawberries)
- 1/4 cup walnuts, chopped
- 1 tbsp flaxseeds, ground
- Honey or maple syrup (optional)

Instructions:

1. In a medium saucepan, bring water or almond milk to a boil. Add oats and a pinch of salt, then reduce the heat to low.

2. Simmer for 5 minutes, stirring occasionally, or until oats are tender and have absorbed most of the liquid.

3. Remove from heat and let sit for two minutes.

4. Stir in ground flaxseeds and sweetener if desired.

5. Serve in bowls topped with fresh berries and walnuts.

As you embark on this culinary journey, let each meal be an opportunity to celebrate the path to a stronger, healthier heart. Remember, embracing heart-healthy habits isn't just about avoidance—it's about discovering the deeply satisfying, delicious foods that also happen to be good for your body. Enjoy these heart-healthy recipes as a cornerstone of your nutrition plan, and feel empowered knowing that you're taking active steps towards a vibrant life filled with vitality.

Appendix C:
Exercise Guides for Every
Fitness Level

Continuing on the path towards a stronger heart and healthier life, let's delve into the practical application of exercise, irrespective of where you are on your fitness journey. This guide is not just about moving; it's about moving right. We understand that each individual's abilities and starting points vary, and that's precisely why we've developed this tailored guide to ensure that no matter your fitness level, there's an exercise routine that can seamlessly blend into your lifestyle, contributing to your heart's vitality.

Getting Started: Foundation of Movement

For those who are new to exercising, or perhaps restarting after a pause or due to health challenges, let's begin by setting a strong foundation. The goal here is not intensity but consistency. Start with short, daily walks, aiming for 5 to 10 minutes at a time. Gradually, as your strength and endurance improve, incrementally increase the duration of your walks. Embrace movement in daily activities, such as taking the stairs instead of the elevator, or parking further away from the store entrance.

Low-Intensity Workouts: Building Stamina

If you have a baseline level of fitness and are ready to elevate your routine, low-intensity workouts will be your next step. Activities such as swimming, cycling on a flat terrain, or gentle yoga not only nurture your heart but are also kind to your joints. Incorporating these activities 3-5 times a week for 20-30 minutes can work wonders in maintaining and improving cardiovascular health.

Moderate-Intensity Exercises: Finding Your Rhythm

Once you've laid the groundwork, stepping up to moderate-intensity exercises will help you find your rhythm. Consider brisk walking, light jogging, or aerobic classes designed to get your heart rate up. These types of exercises are the crux of a well-rounded routine and can significantly enhance heart and lung capacity when performed consistently for at least 30 minutes, 5 days a week.

High-Intensity Training: Challenging Limits

For those who have been actively exercising and are ready for a challenge, high-intensity interval training (HIIT) can yield robust heart health benefits. These workouts alternate between short bursts of intense activity and recovery periods. It's crucial to listen to your body during these exercises, ensuring your heart rate stays within a safe range, especially if you have a history of heart disease or other health concerns.

Strength Training: Bolstering the Musculoskeletal System

Strength training is a powerful ally in maintaining a healthy heart, as it aids in controlling weight, improving metabolism, and reducing the risk of injury by strengthening muscles, tendons, and ligaments. Aim to incorporate strength exercises twice a week, focusing on all major muscle groups. Utilize resistance bands, light weights, or even bodyweight exercises such as push-ups, squats, and lunges to build muscle endurance and support cardiac function.

Stretching and Flexibility: The Cornerstone of Recovery

After each workout session, dedicate time to stretching. Enhancing flexibility not only assists in recovery but also prepares your body for the next exercise session. Including a stretch routine can help mitigate potential soreness and stiffness, making it easier to adhere to a regular exercise regimen.

Remember, the key is to adapt these exercises to your fitness level and progressively challenge your body while ensuring safety. Always consult with your healthcare provider before starting or changing your exercise routine, particularly if you are living with heart disease or other health conditions.

Embarking on a journey to better heart health through exercise isn't just about lowering numbers on a scale or a blood pressure monitor—it's about reclaiming your vitality and enjoying the countless wonders life has to offer. It's about propelling yourself forward with a dynamic spirit, nourishing not just your physical self but also your essence.

Nurturing your heart with appropriate exercise resonates beyond the gym walls—it's an investment in a future where every beat of your heart sings a story of strength, resilience, and unwavering courage. All it takes is the determination to start, the persistence to continue, and the belief that every step you take is a step towards a healthier, heartier you.

Glossary of Heart Health Terms

Embarking on a journey toward better heart health can feel over-whelming with medical jargon that seems foreboding and complex. This glossary is tailored to deconstruct that language barrier, translating key cardiac health terms into digestible explanations. As we navigate deeper into understanding heart health, this glossary will serve as a trusted guide, clarifying the verbiage you'll come across along your path to wellness.

A

- **Angina:** A symptom indicating pain or discomfort in the chest that happens due to reduced blood flow to the heart muscle. It's often a warning sign of underlying heart disease.

- **Atherosclerosis:** The buildup of fats, cholesterol, and other substances in and on your artery walls, which can restrict blood flow.

- **Arrhythmia:** An irregular heartbeat. The heart may beat too fast, too slow, or in an irregular pattern.

B

- **Blood Pressure:** The force of blood pushing against the walls of the arteries. High blood pressure can increase the risk of heart attack and stroke.

- **Body Mass Index (BMI):** A measure of body fat based on height and weight that applies to adult men and women.

C

- **Cardiovascular:** Pertaining to the heart and blood vessels.

- **Cholesterol:** A waxy substance found in blood. High levels of bad cholesterol (LDL) can increase the risk of heart disease and stroke.

D

- **Diabetes:** A chronic condition that affects how your body turns food into energy. It increases the risk of heart disease and stroke.

- **Dyslipidemia:** An abnormal amount of lipids in the blood, increasing the risk of atherosclerosis.

E

- **Echocardiogram:** A test that uses ultrasound to create images of the heart to assess its structure and function.

H

- **Heart Attack (Myocardial Infarction):** An event where blood flow to the heart muscle is severely reduced or stopped, causing tissue damage or death.

- **Heart Failure:** A condition in which the heart can't pump enough blood to meet the body's needs.

- **Hypertension:** Another term for high blood pressure.

M

- **Metabolic Syndrome:** A cluster of conditions that increase the risk of heart disease, stroke, and diabetes. These include increased blood pressure, high blood sugar, excess body fat around the waist, and abnormal cholesterol levels.

- **Murmur:** An unusual sound heard between heartbeats, sometimes indicative of a heart problem.

P

- **Peripheral Artery Disease (PAD):** A condition characterized by narrowed arteries reducing blood flow to the limbs, which can lead to heart disease.

- **Plaque:** A substance made of fat, cholesterol, and other materials, which can build up in the walls of arteries and restrict blood flow.

S

- **Statins:** A class of drugs used to lower blood cholesterol levels by blocking liver substances necessary for making cholesterol.

- **Stroke:** A sudden interruption of blood flow to the brain, caused by a blockage or bursting of a blood vessel, which can result in loss of neurological function.

T

- **Triglycerides:** A type of fat found in blood. High levels can increase the risk of coronary artery disease, especially in women.

This glossary isn't exhaustive; it's a starting point to understanding the language of heart health. With each term you master, you're taking control, not only of your vocabulary but of your well-being. And remember, heart health isn't merely about the absence of disease – it's about choice. The choice to embrace a lifestyle that builds vitality, enhances longevity, and radiates positivity from within.

In mastery of terms and understanding of conditions, you hold the power to engage in informed discussions with your healthcare providers. To make lifestyle choices that don't merely prevent disease but nourish a life rich with experiences you cherish. Your very heartbeat, the pulse echoing through these terms, is your drum of empowerment, echoing a rhythm that speaks of life, resilience, and hope.

As you traverse further chapters and ultimately wield this knowledge as a tool for change, let each newfound concept fortify your heart-smart journey. With every healthier choice, informed decision, and step towards better health, you pave a path for your heart that is as robust as the spirit that drives you.

Made in the USA
Columbia, SC
26 March 2025

55716063R00074